Respiratory Physiology

Basics and Applications

Respiratory Physiology
Basics and Applications

Alan R. Leff, M.D.

Chief • Section of Pulmonary and Critical Care Medicine • Professor of Medicine, Anesthesia and Critical Care • Committee on Cell Physiology and Clinical Pharmacology • Division of the Biological Sciences • University of Chicago • Chicago, Illinois

Paul T. Schumacker, Ph.D

Associate Professor • Department of Medicine and the College • Section of Pulmonary and Critical Care Medicine • Division of Biological Sciences • University of Chicago • Chicago, Illinois

W. B. SAUNDERS COMPANY

A Division of Harcourt Brace & Company

Philadelphia   London   Toronto

Montreal   Sydney   Tokyo

W. B. Saunders Company
A Division of Harcourt Brace & Company

The Curtis Center
Independence Square West
Philadelphia, Pennsylvania 19106

Library of Congress Cataloging-in-Publication Data

Leff, Alan R.
  Respiratory physiology: basics and applications/Alan R. Leff and
Paul T. Schumacker. — 1st ed.
      p. cm.
  Includes index.
  ISBN 0-7216-3952-6
    1. Lungs — Physiology.   2. Lungs — Cytology. I. Schumacker, Paul T.   II. Title.
    [DNLM: 1. Lung — physiology.   2. Lung — cytology.   WF 600 L489r 1993]
QP121.L35 1993
612.2 — dc20
DNLM/DLC   93-6718

Respiratory Physiology: Basics and Applications   ISBN 0-7216-3952-6

Printed in the United States of America.

Last digit is the print number: 9   8   7   6   5   4   3   2   1

DEDICATION

*To our Students at the University of Chicago,
who taught us how to write this book.*

Preface

Medical education is an evolving process. The past decade has revolutionized both clinical and laboratory assessment of lung function and physiology of the lung. Technological advances have made the previously time-consuming process of clinical pulmonary function testing much less arduous. As a result, these data are now used widely by physicians in many specialities in assessing the lung function of their patients.

A particular emphasis of *Respiratory Physiology: Basics and Applications* is not only to present the biophysical and physiological concepts that underlie modern pulmonary physiology and pathophysiology but also to acquaint the reader with their direct application to clinical testing. Whenever possible, examples are drawn from clinical disease states to illustrate physiological principles, and considerable attention has been devoted to the methods by which these physiological measurements are made in patients. A chapter on cardiopulmonary exercise testing is included that integrates physiological concepts developed in the preceding chapters with current methods for breath-by-breath measurements of dynamic lung function.

Through 13 years of teaching the course in respiratory physiology to medical and graduate students in biological science, we have listened to their concerns regarding the balance and content of material that is essential to their knowledge base in clinical and basic science study. A fundamental knowledge of organ physiology and biochemistry is still the central framework on which the physician evaluates lung function. However, the next generation holds forth the promise of innovative therapies emanating from the study of lung cellular and molecular biology. Accordingly, a major component of this text has been devoted to lung growth and development, cellular defense mechanisms in the lung, the neurobiology of the lung, and the biology of conducting airways and their cellular constituents.

In preparing this text, we are most of all grateful to our students, whose comments over the years led to the development of a course syllabus that constituted the framework from which this text was constructed. We wish to thank colleagues who have taken time to review chapters of the text and offer advice, including Dr. Brian Whipp, University of California, Los Angeles (Harbor General Hospital), and Dr. Julian Solway, University of Chicago. We also wish to thank our publisher, W. B. Saunders Company, for faithful and expeditious support in this project.

It is our hope that this text will meet the challenge of providing a balanced presentation of physiological, biochemical, and cell biological science that will meet the educational needs of our medical and graduate students. We also believe that the material may be helpful to both fellows and scholars of respiratory physiology and biology at more advanced levels. It is for students of respiratory science everywhere that this text is written.

Alan R. Leff, M.D.
Paul T. Schumacker, Ph.D.

Contents

Part I

Physiological Functions of the Lung

Chapter 1

Lung Mechanics: Statics

Lung mechanics is the study of the mechanical properties of the lung and chest wall. In the study of lung mechanics, the principles of Newtonian mechanics are applied to the system components. *Lung statics* refers to the mechanical properties of a lung whose volume is not changing with time. Knowledge of the static properties of the respiratory system requires the study of the individual characteristics of the lung and the chest wall. Interaction between the lung and the chest wall is an important determinant of lung volumes, which have important consequences for the gas exchange function of the lung.

DEFINITIONS

Lung volumes are all subdivisions of the *total lung capacity* (TLC). The TLC is the amount of gas con-

tained in the lung at the end of a maximal inspiration (Figure 1–1). All other lung volumes are contained with the TLC either as *volumes* (e.g., the *expiratory reserve volume*) or as *capacities* (e.g., the *functional residual capacity*). A capacity always contains two or more lung volumes. For example, the *inspiratory capacity* is the sum of the *inspiratory reserve volume* plus the *tidal volume*. The understanding of lung mechanics requires a working knowledge of these volumes, for this is the language of lung mechanics.

The *vital capacity* (VC) is the maximum amount of air that can be exhaled from the lung after inspiration to TLC. The VC consists of the *inspiratory capacity* (IC), which is the maximum amount of gas that can be inspired from the resting end-expiratory lung volume, plus the *expiratory reserve volume* (ERV), which is the maximum volume of gas that

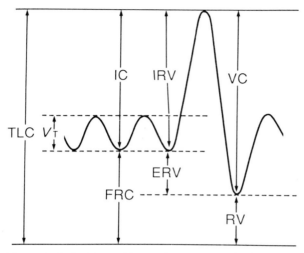

Figure 1–1. Divisions of lung volumes as inscribed by a spirometer: TLC, total lung capacity; IC, inspiratory capacity; IRV, inspiratory reserve volume; FRC, functional residual capacity; ERV, expiratory reserve volume; VC, vital capacity; RV, residual volume; Vт, tidal volume. (From Brewis RAL, Gibson GJ, Geddes DM [eds]: Respiratory Medicine London, Baillière Tindall, 1990.)

can be exhaled from the end of a passive exhalation. The IC is further divided into the *inspiratory reserve volume* (IRV), which is the maximum volume of gas that can be inspired beginning at the end of a normal inspiration, and the *tidal volume* (Vт), which is the volume of gas that moves in and out of the lungs during normal breathing.

The *functional residual capacity* (FRC) is the volume of gas remaining in the lungs at the end of a passive expiration. The FRC is normally determined by a balance between the tendency of the chest wall to expand outward and the opposing tendency of the lung to collapse to a smaller lung volume (see later). Some amount of air always remains within the lung, even after a maximal exhalation. This volume, the *residual volume* (RV), is the amount of gas remaining in the lung after a maximal expiratory effort.

MEASUREMENT OF LUNG VOLUMES

One method used to measure lung volumes is *spirometry*. In patients undergoing pulmonary function testing, the relationship of their measured lung volumes to expected normal values forms the

basis of clinical pulmonary function testing. The spirometer is an instrument used for measuring most lung volumes. Although there are many varieties of spirometers, the classic *water seal spirometer* is shown in Figure 1–2. This spirometer is an air-filled container constructed from two cylinders (drums) of different size. The larger cylinder contains a water-filled sleeve, and the smaller cylinder is inverted and suspended in this sleeve from a pulley. The water provides a seal that prevents the escape of gas. A counterweight balances the inverted cylinder, and a pen attached to the weight records the motion of the floating drum. As the patient breathes through the mouthpiece, gas enters or leaves the inside of the floating cylinder. As air is withdrawn from the cylinder the counterbalance weight moves upward, producing an upward tracing of the pen. Conversely, during exhalation a downward tracing is produced. The rotation of the recording drum spreads out the display, so that the pen tracings are not recorded on top of each other. If the recording drum rotates at constant speed, the abscissa will represent *time.* Thus, the y-axis is a measure of the change in lung volume and the x-axis represents time. This makes it possible to assess flow rates from the slope of the line generated, because flow is the rate of change of volume with respect to time ($\Delta V / \Delta t$). A subject breathing from a spirometer can generate a tracing like that shown in Figure 1–1.

With the use of the spirometer tracing shown in Figure 1–1, some general relationships among lung and volumes/capacities can be noted. The Vт is normally 400 to 500 ml, and FRC is achieved reproducibly at the end of each Vт. The VC is normally about 75% of TLC. However, some relationships cannot be obtained from the spirometer because it only measures lung volumes above RV. Because the spirometer cannot measure how much gas remains in the lung after a maximal exhalation (RV), it cannot be used to measure TLC or FRC directly. Hence, an alternative method must be used to measure TLC, FRC, or RV.

One method of measuring total lung capacity is the *gas dilution technique.* By this method, the subject inspires a trace concentration of an inert gas (such as helium). The gas must be nontoxic (to protect the patient) and highly insoluble in blood (to minimize absorption into the blood). The patient inspires the tracer gas mixture to TLC and performs

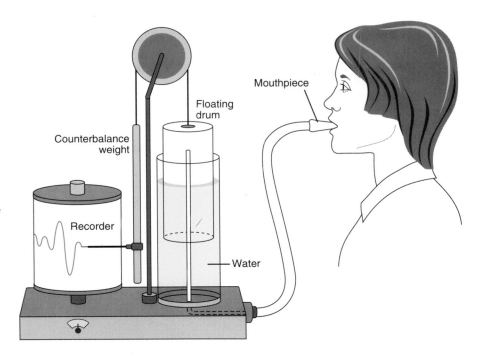

Figure 1-2. A classic water seal spirometer. The kymograph is rotated so that the spirogram, as shown in Figure 1-1, is inscribed. Volumes are recorded on the *y*-axis against time on the *x*-axis.

a 10-second breath-holding maneuver. The patient then exhales, and the concentration of helium is measured by an analyzer that samples gas from the mouthpiece. (The sample is taken from the mid-expiration to be certain that it is representative of fully mixed gas.) The average exhaled concentration of the tracer will be less than the inhaled concentration because it is diluted by the volume of gas present in the lungs at the start of inhalation (e.g., FRC). By conservation of mass, the product of tracer concentration and volume of gas containing the tracer remains constant. Hence,

$$C_1 V_1 = C_2 V_2$$

where C_1 and V_1 are the inhaled tracer concentration and inhaled volume of gas, C_2 is the exhaled (diluted) tracer concentration, and V_2 is the total volume of distribution of the tracer (TLC). Because C_1 is known and V_1 and C_2 can be measured, V_2 can be calculated. This volume, V_2, is the TLC.

$$V_2 = C_1 V_1 / C_2$$

$$V_2 = TLC$$

Although this technique provides a measure of the

TLC, it has limitations in patients with certain forms of lung disease. In some lung diseases, patients have lung regions that contain gas but into which little or no fresh gas enters. If the tracer gas fails to reach these airspaces in the lung during the breath-holding period, the concentration of helium measured during exhalation (C_2) will be greater than it would have been if there were uniform distribution of gas throughout the lung. Accordingly, the TLC measured by this method will underestimate the true TLC.

This problem is particularly common in patients with *chronic obstructive pulmonary disease* and *asthma* because large regions of the lung may receive very little ventilation compared with other areas. To ensure accurate measurement of TLC, FRC, and RV in these patients it is necessary to employ a method that does not depend on the *distribution of ventilation* within the lung.

BODY PLETHYSMOGRAPHY

Lung volumes can be measured most accurately in the *body plethysmograph* (Figure 1-3), also known as the *body box*. This device is an airtight chamber

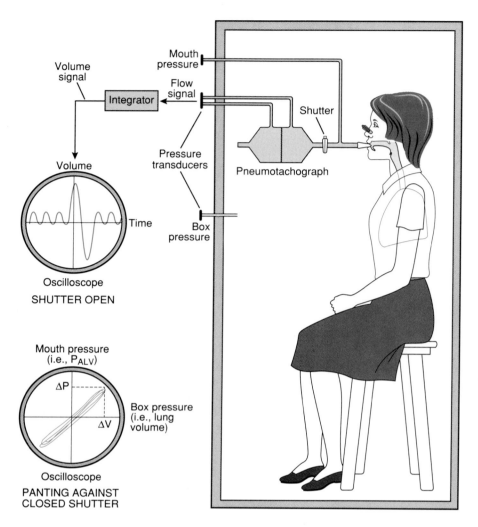

Figure 1–3. Diagram of body plethysmograph. This instrument measures both lung volume and airway resistance (see Chapter 2). Box pressure transducer measures change in lung volume while panting (see text), and mouth pressure transducer measures pressure in the lung at zero flow when the shutter is closed. Recordings of box and mouth pressures are made on an oscilloscope, and the resulting angle (y vs. x) is obtained as shown. This angle X atmospheric pressure measures the volume at which the patient is panting, which is the functional residual capacity.

in which the patient sits while breathing through a mouthpiece. Use of a nose clip ensures that the patient breathes only through the mouthpiece. The body plethysmograph operates on the principle of Boyle's law, applied to the volume of gas in the lungs. Boyle's law states that the product of pressure and volume for a gas in a chamber is constant, under isothermal conditions. Thus,

$$P \cdot V = k$$

where P is pressure and V is volume in a closed system.

The pressure inside the plethysmograph (the box) remains constant as the patient inhales because the total volume of gas in the box does not change. While the patient sits in the box, several tidal volumes are observed. As the patient breathes, the flow of gas (ml/min) through the mouthpiece is measured using a *flow transducer (pneumotachograph)*. The V_T volume (ml) can be determined by electronically integrating the inspired flow signal obtained from the pneumotachograph (see Figure 1–3) (volume vs. time). The plot of V_T as a function of time yields a spirogram similar to that shown in Figure 1–1, and FRC is easily observed at the end of each breath. A *shutter* (normally open) near the mouthpiece is closed at FRC, and the patient is asked to pant rapidly (two to three times per second) against the closed shutter. Because the shutter is closed there is no airflow in the system and air is compressed and decompressed in the lungs. A pressure transducer attached to the mouthpiece is used to record the pressure at the mouth. If isothermal conditions during this procedure are assumed, the following relationship holds:

$$V_1 \cdot P_1 = V_2 \cdot P_2$$

where V_1 is the lung volume when the shutter is closed (FRC), P_1 is the mouth pressure when the shutter is closed (i.e., atmospheric), and V_2 and P_2 are the lung volume and mouth pressure during the attempted exhalation. This relationship can be rearranged to yield the following:

$$FRC \cdot P_{FRC} = (FRC + \Delta V)(P_{FRC} + \Delta P)$$

where FRC is the starting lung volume and P_{FRC} is the pressure in the airway at FRC (atmospheric). The ΔV and ΔP terms represent the changes in lung volume and airway (mouth) pressure produced during the panting maneuver. The right side of the equation represents the product of volume and pressure that must remain constant during the panting maneuver (i.e., greater or less than the volume and pressure at FRC but always having the same product). This is an expression of Boyle's law. Rearranging terms to solve for the FRC volume,

$$FRC \cdot P_{FRC} = FRC \cdot P_{FRC} + P_{FRC} \cdot \Delta V$$
$$+ FRC \cdot \Delta P + \Delta P \cdot \Delta V.$$

Compared with the value of P_{FRC} (which is atmospheric pressure) and FRC (normally about 3 liters), ΔV (30 ml) and ΔP (20 cm H_2O) are small. Hence, $\Delta V \cdot \Delta P$ is a very small value indeed and can be ignored without introducing a large error. Thus, the equation can now be written as

$$FRC \cdot P_{FRC} = FRC \cdot P_{FRC} + P_{FRC} \cdot \Delta V$$
$$+ FRC \cdot \Delta P.$$

Subtracting $FRC \cdot P_{FRC}$ from both sides

$$- P_{FRC} \cdot \Delta V = FRC \cdot \Delta P$$

or

$$FRC = P_{FRC} \cdot \frac{\Delta V}{\Delta P}$$

Note that the minus sign is dropped, since it has no

physiological significance. Recall that P_{FRC} is the pressure in the airways when the shutter was closed (atmospheric). Hence,

$$FRC = P_{atmospheric} \cdot \frac{\Delta V}{\Delta P}$$

Thus, to measure FRC using the body box one needs to measure the ratio of $\Delta V / \Delta P$ during panting and the atmospheric pressure (which can be obtained from a barometer). Because the subject pants rapidly (two to three times per second), the volume and pressure signals change rapidly. Hence, it is advisable to use instruments that can faithfully record rapidly changing events, such as an oscilloscope. By convention, box pressure is recorded on the y-axis (see Figure 1–3).

Note that because pressure measurements at the mouth are made with the shutter closed, virtually no airflow occurs in the airways during panting. Consequently, the pressure in the mouth is the same as the pressure in the lung alveoli during the panting maneuver. By analogy, consider a fireplace bellows whose orifice is plugged by a cork. When the bellows is squeezed or expanded, the pressure everywhere in the bellows increases and decreases equally (and can be measured at the spout). By contrast, if the cork is removed and air is expelled from the bellows the pressure at the spout is less than the pressure within the bellows. Thus, pressure in the alveoli can be obtained by measuring pressure at the mouthpiece. By convention this is recorded as a vertical deflection on the y-axis during panting.

Normally, the changes in lung volume (ΔV) that occur during panting against a closed shutter are recorded on the x-axis. In practice, the changes in volume are usually obtained from the measured changes in pressure within the body box. As the lungs expand, air is compressed in the box, causing an increase in pressure that is measured with a pressure transducer. Because Boyle's law applies to the gas sealed within the box, the changes in lung volume during panting are proportional to the pressure changes measured in the box. Thus, the lung volume changes during panting can be calculated from the box pressure changes if the relationship between ΔP and ΔV for the gas in the box is known. This relationship (the *body box calibration*) can be obtained by applying a known volume change to the box (using a piston or syringe) and measuring the change in pressure while the subject is seated inside.

Because all gas within the chest is compressed and expanded during the panting maneuver, the value of FRC obtained from the body plethysmograph measures the total thoracic gas volume at FRC, even if it is trapped beyond an obstructed airway. Since this method does not depend on tracer gas equilibration in all lung regions, it is the preferred method for measuring lung volumes in patients with advanced lung disease. To determine TLC, the inspiratory capacity (determined from standard spirometry) is added to FRC obtained from the body box. In principle, the body box could thus be used to measure any lung volume directly. FRC is normally chosen because it is highly reproducible and comfortable for panting. (Try panting at TLC!)

A third method to determine lung volume is extremely accurate and is not affected by disease states of the lung. This is the method of *radiographic planimetry*. For this, chest roentgenograms are obtained in the anteroposterior and lateral projections (front and side) and a calibrated instrument called a *planimeter* is used to outline the dimensions of the lung. Although accurate, this method is inconvenient, expensive, and only rarely used.

DETERMINANTS OF LUNG VOLUME

From both a physiological and clinical perspective it is important to be able to measure lung volumes, especially TLC, because these values reflect the physical properties of the lung and help to diagnose disease states. To understand what factors influence lung volumes that are altered in health and disease, it is useful to begin by examining the normal determinants of lung volume.

Pulmonary Compliance

Compliance is a physical term that relates change in the volume of a closed system to the change in the pressure distending it. A lung with a *high compliance* is one that is easily distended. A lung with a *reduced compliance* is one that is difficult to distend. Given the same distending pressure, a lung with a high compliance will reach a higher volume than a lung

with a decreased compliance. Compliance is the mathematical inverse of *elastance*. Hence, a lung with high elastance is one that is difficult to distend —a *stiff* lung.

Pulmonary compliance (C_L) is equal to the change in volume per unit change in distending pressure, or

$$C_L = \Delta V \text{ (in liters)}/\Delta P \text{ (in cm } H_2O).$$

Thus, the units of compliance are liters/cm H_2O. The value obtained for compliance of a given lung depends on the volume of that lung. As shown in Figure 1–4, if a 5 cm H_2O increase in pressure is required to increase the volume of lungs R + L by 1 liter, the compliance will be 1.0 liter/5 cm H_2O. For situation 1,

$$C_L = 1.0 \text{ liter}/5 \text{ cm } H_2O$$

$$= 0.2 \text{ liter/cm } H_2O.$$

Next consider the situation in which lung R has been removed. Application of 5 cm H_2O distending pressure now will distend lung L by the same amount as before (situation 2), but the total lung volume change will be only half of what is was when both lungs were present. In this situation

$$C_L = 0.5 \text{ liter}/5 \text{ cm } H_2O$$

$$= 0.1 \text{ liter/cm } H_2O.$$

Situation 3 details an extreme case in which lung R is removed and much of lung L has also been resected. The value obtained in this situation is much smaller than when lung volume was larger, even though the intrinsic elastic character of the lung tissue has not been changed. Thus, the value obtained for C_L is dependent on the lung volume. As shown in Figure 1–4, volume-related differences in compliance can be *normalized* by dividing the compliance by the FRC. This value is termed the *specific compliance*. Note in the above example that the specific compliance remained constant because the distensibility of a given amount of lung tissue was unaltered in all three situations. This normalization provides a measure of the elastic properties of the lung tissue, lest compliance in the smaller individ-

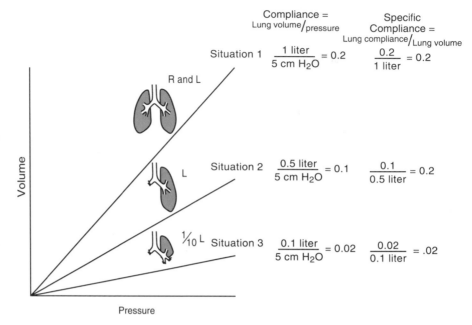

Figure 1–4. Relationship between lung compliance and lung volume. Because compliance is a volume-dependent measurement, lung excision will reduce compliance, even though the elastic properties of the lung remain unchanged. By dividing by the functional residual capacity to obtain specific compliance, all values are equalized. (Adapted and redrawn from Comroe JH: Physiology of Respiration, 2nd ed. Chicago, Year Book Medical Publishers, 1975.)

ual be penalized by the smaller lung volume at FRC (Figure 1–5).

In measuring the compliance of a system, the pressure term represents the *transmural pressure difference,* that is, the inside-minus-outside pressure difference. Thus, ΔP represents a *change* in the transmural (distending) pressure. Note that the compliance of the respiratory system (lungs plus chest wall) can be measured by progressively inflating the lungs with a positive pressure while measuring the difference between airway and atmospheric pressure (inside − outside).

Lung-Chest Wall Interactions

The lung and chest wall act together but are separated by the *pleural space.* The pleural space should be thought of as a potential space, since the volume separating parietal and visceral pleura of the lung is very small under normal conditions. Thus, changes in the volume of the lung and the chest wall are equal under intact conditions. The transmural pressure for the lung *(transpulmonary pressure)* is defined as the pressure difference between the airspaces of the lung (alveolar pressure) and the pressure

surrounding the lung (pleural pressure). The lung requires a positive transmural pressure to increase its volume above RV, much like a latex balloon. As the transmural distending pressure is increased (going from RV to TLC), the lung volume increases. Unlike the chest wall, the lung will contract to a very small *minimal volume* if the transmural distending pressure decreases to zero. Thus, C_L can be measured if the lung is inflated in a stepwise manner while the transpulmonary pressure is measured. Note that the C_L *alone* can be determined if the difference in pressure between the airways and the pleural space measured while the lung is progressively inflated.

The chest wall is an elastic container that tends to expand (spring out) to a larger volume than it assumes during quiet breathing. During normal breathing the pressure in the pleural space is negative with respect to atmospheric pressure. This produces a negative transmural pressure for the chest wall, which keeps the chest wall pulled in to a smaller volume during normal breathing. If the chest is surgically opened to the atmosphere, the transmural pressure for the lung and chest wall decrease to zero. In this situation the lung and chest wall will become separated from each other as the

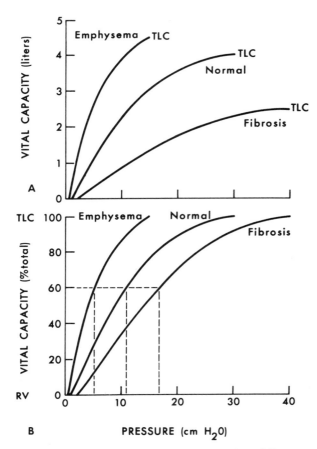

Figure 1–5. Schematic compliance curves in three different states: emphysema, normal lung, and lung with pulmonary fibrosis. *Top.* Because lungs with pulmonary fibrosis have low lung volumes to begin with (the scar tissue constricts the lung) and patients with emphysema (lungs have lost elastic tissue) have larger than normal lung volumes, there is a volume-dependent spread of these compliance curves. *Bottom.* By correcting for lung volume (expressing the ordinate as a percentage of the vital capacity), these curves come closer together, but it still can be noted that the fibrotic lung is stiffer and the lung with emphysema is more compliant than a normal lung. (From Murray JF: The Normal Lung, 2nd ed. Philadelphia, WB Saunders, 1986.)

sealed and studied. The chest wall and lung curve would be obtained by studying an intact subject. In each case, the curves are obtained by passively inflating the lungs (and/or the chest wall) with a large syringe. The volume of each structure is plotted as a function of the respective transmural (inside − outside) distending pressure. (Note that if the pressure outside is zero [atmospheric], the transmural pressure is merely the inside pressure.)

Consider the properties of the chest wall alone. When the pressure in the chest is opened to the atmosphere, the transmural pressure decreases to zero, and the chest wall assumes a volume of approximately 60% of TLC. If gas is removed from the chest, the transmural pressure becomes negative and the chest volume decreases. At a transmural pressure of about −40 cm H_2O, the chest wall reaches RV. If gas is pumped into the chest, the volume reaches TLC when the transmural pressure is approximately 10 cm H_2O.

Next, consider the pressure–volume relationship for the lung alone. If the airway is opened to the atmosphere, the lung transmural pressure decreases to zero and the lung will be at its minimal volume, which is less than RV (not shown). If gas is pumped into the lung, the transmural pressure increases. At a lung transmural pressure of 10 cm H_2O, the lung volume will be approximately 50% of TLC, and TLC will be reached when the lung transmural pressure reaches 30 cm H_2O.

The pressure–volume relationship for the intact system reflects the algebraic sum of the pressures exerted by the lung and the chest wall. At RV, the lung is very minimally distended, and it contributes little to the combined pressures in the lung–chest wall system. The properties of the intact system at this volume are essentially those of the chest wall alone at RV. Under normal conditions, RV is determined by the ability of the expiratory muscles to develop a sufficiently negative distending pressure to oppose the outward recoil forces of the chest wall. As the chest wall is squeezed by the expiratory muscles to progressively lower volumes, the recoil pressure of the chest wall increases. However, ability of the expiratory muscles to generate force also decreases as the muscles shorten. Residual volume therefore is set by the balance between (1) diminishing expiratory muscle force generation at low lung volumes and (2) increasing chest wall recoil at low lung volumes (point A, see Figure 1–6).

The transmural pressure for the intact system can

chest wall expands to a larger volume and the lung collapses to a smaller volume.

Figure 1–6 demonstrates the *pressure–volume relationships* for the lung alone, the chest wall alone, and the intact system (lungs plus chest wall) acting together. The curve representing the lung alone would be obtained if the lungs were removed from the chest and inflated separately. The curve for the chest wall alone would be obtained if the lungs were removed from the chest and the chest wall was re-

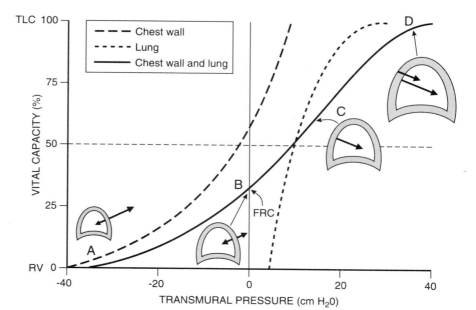

Figure 1-6. The lung–chest wall system. *A.* At residual volume. *B.* At functional residual capacity. *C.* At the natural resting volume of the chest wall. *D.* At a volume near total lung capacity. (Redrawn from Murray JF: The Normal Lung, 2nd ed. Philadelphia, WB Saunders, 1986.)

be reduced to zero if the airways are opened to the atmosphere. This is precisely the situation at the end of a passive exhalation when the glottis is open and the lung is at FRC (point B, see Figure 1 – 6). Here the transmural pressure for the chest wall is approximately -7.5 cm H_2O and the lung transmural pressure is $+7.5$ cm H_2O. Thus, the tendency of the chest wall to recoil to a larger volume is equal to the tendency of the lung to collapse to a smaller volume. This equilibrium determines the FRC. This equilibrium point is highly reproducible because it is determined entirely by the balance between the opposing pressure–volume properties of the lung and chest wall. [Note that neither the inspiratory nor the expiratory muscles are working at FRC.]

When the volume of the intact system is at about 60% of VC, the transmural pressure of the chest wall is nearly zero, so the chest wall contributes little to the behavior of the whole system. Thus, at this volume the recoil properties of the lung–chest wall system are determined essentially by the lung itself (point C). There is no particular term for this volume.

At volumes greater than 60% of VC, both the lung and chest wall require positive transmural distending pressures (point D). Consequently, at these higher volumes the lung and chest wall contribute additively to the effective recoil of the system,

which exceeds that of either the lung or the chest wall alone. When the transmural distending pressure for the lung exceeds approximately 20 cm H_2O, the pressure–volume curve of the lung tends to "flatten." Thus, further increases in distending pressure do not cause significant increases in lung volume. In this region, the lung compliance is less because the elastic limits of the lung as a distensible organ are being reached. At this point, the connective tissue of the lung (e.g., collagen, elastin) limits further distention. Attempts to inflate the lung further may produce a rupture of the visceral pleura, allowing air to escape from the lung into the pleural space *(pneumothorax).* [Development of pneumothorax is a significant clinical complication in patients with stiff lungs who are mechanically ventilated with a positive-pressure ventilator. The high distending pressures required to inflate a lung with reduced compliance may exceed the elastic limit of the lung tissue or airways.]

What determines the TLC? The TLC is determined by the balance between the ability of the inspiratory muscles to increase the lung–chest wall system and the recoil forces generated by the system at high volumes. At higher lung volumes the inspiratory muscles shorten progressively, and their ability to generate force decreases. The volume at which recoil of the lung–chest wall system is balanced by

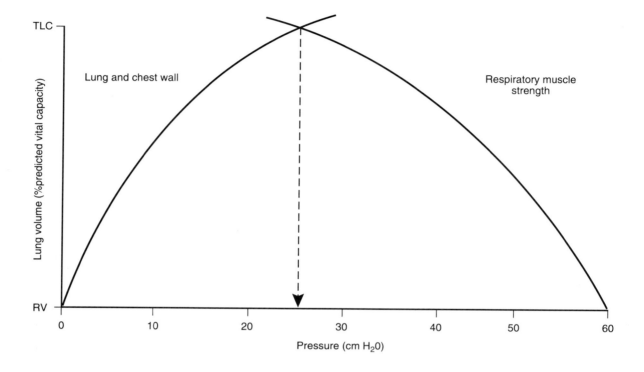

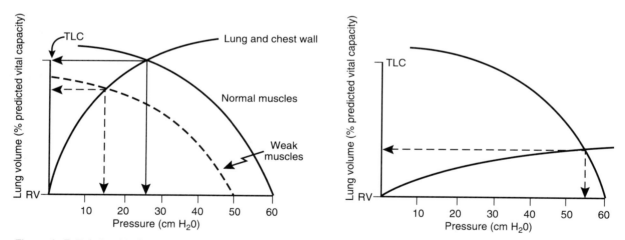

Figure 1–7. Relationship between the lung–chest wall system and the respiratory muscles. Total lung capacity (TLC) is determined by the ability of the chest wall muscles to oppose the recoil of the lung and chest wall. In this drawing, chest wall recoil is assumed to be normal in all three examples. At higher volumes, recoil increases and muscle strength decreases (with progressive shortening). *Top.* TLC is determined where these two factors balance. *Bottom left.* Effect of respiratory muscle weakness. There is a shift to left of muscle curve, and TLC is decreased, as is the maximal elastic recoil pressure. *Bottom right.* Effect of increased lung elastance (e.g., pulmonary fibrosis). The stiff lung has a flat pressure–volume curve, which causes a low TLC but a *high* maximum elastic recoil pressure. (Redrawn from Gibson GJ, Pride NJ: Lung distensibility. Br J Dis Chest 70:143–183, 1976.)

the ability of inspiratory muscles to generate distending force is the TLC. This point is illustrated in Figure 1–7. Under some conditions the respiratory muscles may become weak. For example, in diseases of the musculoskeletal system such as myasthenia gravis, glycogen storage diseases, muscular dystrophy, and multiple sclerosis, the maximum force generated by the respiratory muscles is impaired. In these diseases, the pressure–volume curve generated by the respiratory muscles, which has the inverse contour of that for the lung–chest wall system (see Figure 1–6), shifts to the left (see Figure 1–7). The net result is a lower TLC even though the intrinsic pressure–volume relationship for the respiratory system is normal.

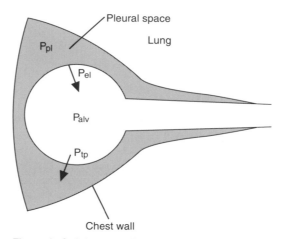

Figure 1–8. Schematic of the relationship between the pleural, alveolar, and elastic recoil pressures of the lung. (Redrawn from Gibson GJ, Pride NJ: Lung distensibility. Br J Dis Chest 70:143–183, 1976.)

LUNG DISTENSIBILITY

Transpulmonary Pressure

For diagnostic purposes, it is desirable to be able to assess the elastic properties of lung independently from those of the chest wall or lung–chest wall system. To do this, it is necessary to measure the transmural distending pressure across the lung alone, excluding the chest wall. The transmural pressure for the lung alone is termed the *transpulmonary pressure* (P_{tp}). It is the pressure difference between the alveoli and the pleural space (transpulmonary = across the lung pleura, that is, from the alveolus to the pleura) (Figure 1–8). Under static conditions, P_{tp} determines the volume of the lung. Accordingly,

$$P_{tp} = \text{(pressure in the alveolus)}$$

$$- \text{(pleural pressure)}.$$

Symbolically,

$$P_{tp} = P_{alv} - P_{pl}.$$

Because the alveoli are not rigid, any pressure change in the pleural space (positive or negative) will be transmitted through the pleural surface into the alveoli. (This would not be the case if the lung was totally rigid, like a hollow steel ball, for exam-

ple.) Accordingly,

$$P_{alv} = P_{el} + P_{pl}$$

where P_{el} is the static recoil pressure generated by the lung and P_{alv} is the gas pressure inside the alveoli. For example, at FRC the elastic recoil pressure of the lung (7.5 cm H_2O) is balanced exactly by the chest wall recoil pressure, which is -7.5 cm H_2O:

$$P_{alv} = 7.5 \text{ cm } H_2O + (-7.5 \text{ cm } H_2O) = 0$$

Because the P_{alv} is the same as atmospheric pressure at FRC, air does not flow in or out of the lung when the glottis is open. Substituting from above,

$$P_{el} = P_{alv} - P_{el}.$$

Substituting for P_{el},

$$P_{tp} = P_{alv} - (P_{alv} - P_{el}).$$

Thus,

$$P_{tp} = P_{el}.$$

In practice, P_{tp} may be regarded as the pressure distending the lung, whereas P_{el} may be thought of as the pressure tending to collapse the lung under

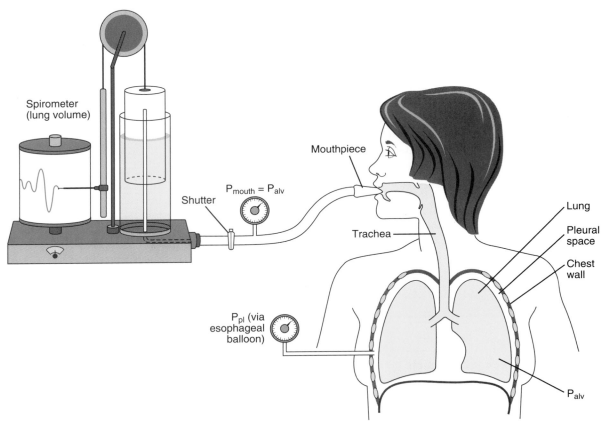

Figure 1-9. An apparatus for measuring the pressure–volume curve of the lung independent of the chest wall. Transpulmonary pressure is measured using a catheter connected to an esophageal balloon.

static conditions (i.e., no flow). For lung volume to remain stable, it is obvious that the distending (transmural) and recoil (P_{el}) pressures must be the same.

The Pressure–Volume Curve of the Lung

The pressure–volume relationships for the lung can be determined by measuring the transpulmonary pressure at different lung volumes. This requires the measurement of pleural pressure, which can be obtained using an *esophageal balloon catheter* in the esophagus. The esophageal balloon catheter is a tube connected to a floppy balloon that is swallowed and positioned in the mid-thoracic esopha-

gus. Because the esophagus is a floppy tube that passes through the thorax, the pressure in the pleural space is transmitted across the esophageal wall into the floppy balloon. A pressure transducer is then connected to the catheter to measure the pressure in the balloon. Alveolar pressure is the same as the pressure in the mouth, as long as the glottis is open and no airflow is occurring.

Lung compliance is measured clinically using the apparatus shown schematically in Figure 1–9. The subject first inspires to TLC, and the shutter is closed. At this lung volume the pressure is measured simultaneously at the mouth and in the pleural space (esophageal balloon). The difference between P_{alv} and P_{pl} yields P_{tp}. For example, at TLC with the glottis open the alveolar pressure is zero while the pleural pressure is about -30 cm H_2O.

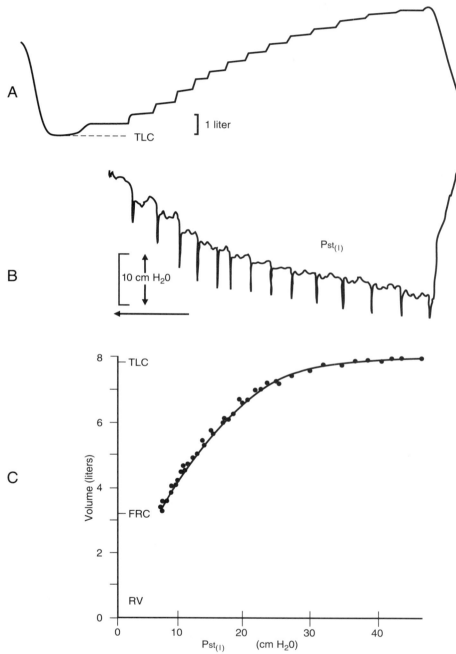

Figure 1–10. Tracing of an actual pressure–volume curve generated during a study of pulmonary compliance. *A:* Spirogram showing change in lung volume from TLC to RV. *B:* corresponding changes in transpulmonary pressure. NB: $P_{st(l)} = P_{tp}$. *C:* Resulting plot of *A* and *B.* (Redrawn from Gibson GJ, Pride NJ: Lung distensibility. Br J Dis Chest 70:143–183, 1976.)

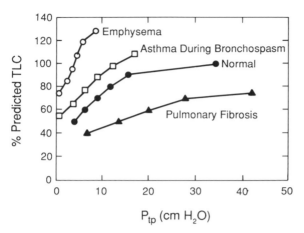

Figure 1–11. Schema of compliance curves in various disease states. Note that volumes are corrected to the predicted total lung capacity of each individual (see Fig. 1–4). The lung in a patient with severe asthma is somewhat hypercompliant; however, the mechanism for this is unknown. (Redrawn from Gibson GJ, Pride NJ: Lung distensibility. Br J Dis Chest 70:143–183, 1976.)

Hence, the transpulmonary pressure can be calculated as

$$P_{tp} = P_{alv} - P_{pl}$$

or

$$P_{tp} = 30 \text{ cm H}_2\text{O} = 0 \text{ cm H}_2\text{O} - (-30 \text{ cm H}_2\text{O}).$$

The shutter is then opened, and the subject exhales to a slightly lower volume, whereon the shutter is closed and a new measurement is made. Normally this process is repeated from TLC to FRC. [At volumes below FRC, pleural pressure measurements are not accurate because mechanical compression of the esophagus by the surrounding mediastinal structures causes the esophageal pressure measurement to deviate from the true pleural pressure.]

Note that if the subject tries to exhale against a closed shutter during the above procedure, the resulting increase in pleural pressure is transmitted across the pleura causing an increase in P_{alv} but leaving P_{tp} unchanged. For example, if the subject increases pleural pressure from −30 cm H$_2$O to 70 cm H$_2$O at TLC by this effort, P_{alv} increases by the same amount (100 cm H$_2$O) but P_{tp} remains the same. Accordingly,

$$P_{tp} = 100 \text{ cm H}_2\text{O} - 70 \text{ cm H}_2\text{O} = 30 \text{ cm H}_2\text{O}.$$

Figure 1–10 shows a pressure–volume curve of the

lung generated by this method. The shape of the lung pressure–volume curve, along with the maximum P_{tp} generated, is useful in describing the pathophysiology of a number of lung diseases. Figure 1–11 shows representative examples of the lung pressure–volume curves found in patients with some common lung abnormalities.

SURFACE TENSION

Figure 1–12 is a drawing of a pressure–volume relationship for an excised lung. When the lungs are inflated and deflated with air, two different curves are obtained. During inflation, a higher transmural pressure is required to achieve any given lung vol-

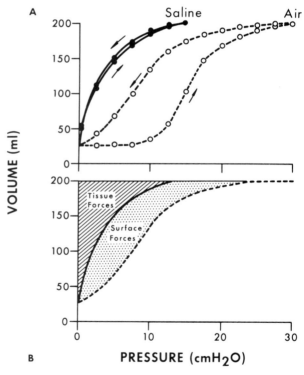

Figure 1–12. Effect of air–water interface of lung distensibility. *Top.* Note hysteresis that is lost as lungs are inflated with saline. *Bottom.* Relative work required to distend lung as a function of surface active force and tissue elastic forces. Dashed line represents the average of the inflation and deflation limbs of the air inflation and deflation curves. (From Clements JA, Tierney DF: Alveolar instability associated with altered surface tension. In Fenn WO, Rahn H [eds]: Handbook of Physiology, Section 3, Respiration, vol. II, pp 1565–1583. Washington, DC, American Physiological Society, 1965.)

ume below TLC compared with deflation. This separation of the inflation and deflation limbs of the pressure–volume curves is termed *hysteresis.* When the same lung is instead inflated with saline, a different pressure–volume relationship is generated that does not demonstrate hysteresis. Note that the C_L is much larger during saline inflation because a smaller increase in distending pressure is required to achieve a given change in lung volume.

The reason for the hysteresis and the differences in compliance that occur with air versus saline inflation relates to surface tension forces that exist in the alveoli. The alveolar surface is lined with a liquid, which forms an air–liquid interface with alveolar gas. Surface tension at the air–liquid interface tends to increase the lung elastic recoil pressure generated at any given lung volume. When the air–liquid interface is abolished by inflating the lung with saline, only the elastic structural elements in the lung tissue contribute to the lung recoil. As shown in Figure 1–12, the surface tension forces contribute substantially to the total lung recoil.

During normal breathing, work is required to increase the lung and chest wall volume from FRC to the end-inspiratory volume. The work to inflate the lung itself reflects the product of the force required to overcome the elastic recoil of the lung and the distance (volume change) over which the force is applied (i.e., pressure $\times$ change in volume). The work performed in overcoming surface forces in the lung during inflation is proportional to the difference in recoil pressure generated by the saline-filled and the air-filled lung during inflation to a given volume (see Figure 1–12, *bottom*). The integrated area to the left of the saline-filled curve represents the work required to overcome the tissue elastic forces in the lung during a full inflation. Note that during exhalation this potential energy is returned as the lung elastic (structural) elements relax. The total area to the left of the dashed line (see Figure 1–12, *bottom*) represents the work required to overcome structural elastic plus surface tension forces during a complete inhalation. Note that during exhalation only part of this potential energy is recovered in deflating the lung because the surface tension forces generated during exhalation are less than during inhalation. The difference between the work expended during inflation and that recovered during deflation represents the work performed on the lung, which is converted to heat. Note that approximately one half of the total work is due to overcoming surface tension forces and one half is attributable to tissue elastic forces. Note also that at FRC (and for the initial volumes above FRC), sur-

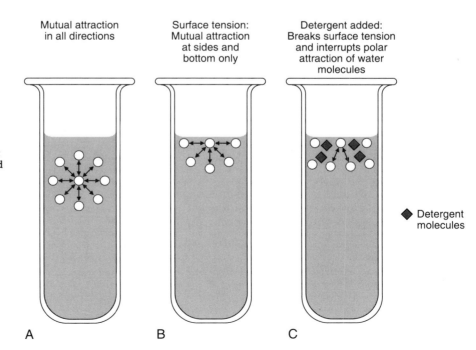

Figure 1–13. Effect of detergent on surface tension. (Adapted and redrawn from Comroe JH: Physiology of Respiration, 2nd ed. Chicago, Year Book Medical Publishers, 1975.)

Mutual attraction in all directions

Surface tension: Mutual attraction at sides and bottom only

Detergent added: Breaks surface tension and interrupts polar attraction of water molecules

◆ Detergent molecules

A   B   C

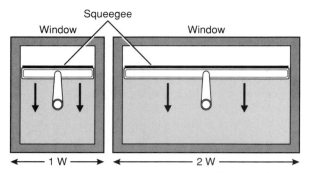

Figure 1–14. Squeegee/window analogy. If a given force is required to pull a squeegee over a windowpane to clean it, a squeegee twice the length will require twice the force. By analogy, tension is a force/length, which is the same in both cases.

face tension is the most important force that must be overcome during inspiration.

Figure 1–13 demonstrates the concept of surface tension. In test tube A, a water molecule below the surface is shown with equal attractive forces surrounding it in all directions. These are the attractive forces created by the polar configuration of the H_2O molecule. The molecule in test tube A is surrounded by other water molecules in three dimensions. The "pull" caused by the attractive forces on the molecule by other water molecules therefore is equivalent in all directions. In test tube B, a molecule is represented at the surface and there is an air–water interface. This molecule is acted on by polar force of other water molecules from beneath it and laterally but not from above (the air interface); this creates a tension (*surface tension*) across the surface of the water. A detergent with a polar and a nonpolar end is added to test tube C. The polar end is attracted to the water molecule, and the nonpolar end interrupts the polar attraction of other water molecules. This reduces the surface tension.

The units of surface tension are those of a force applied per unit length. This can be conceptualized as a window-washing "squeegee," as shown in Figure 1–14. If window B is twice the width of window A, it will require twice the force to clean window B but the same "tension" (force/unit length). This is the normalized force required to move the cleaner (i.e., squeegee) over the window.

Surface tension is a measure of the attractive force of the surface molecules per unit length of the ma-terial to which they are attracted. A *Maxwell frame* can be used to measure surface tension (Figure 1–15A). First, the sliding bar of the frame is dragged across the frame, and the frictional force is calculated and divided by the length of the bar. Next the frame is filled with a liquid for which the surface tension is to be measured. It is filled precisely to the level of the blade so that a monolayer of molecules adheres to the blade. Then the blade is again dragged across the frame. The force/length of the second maneuver exceeds that from the first maneuver (no fluid) by the amount equal to the surface tension.

$$\text{Surface tension} = \frac{(\text{force}_{\text{after fluid}} - \text{force}_{\text{initial}})}{\text{blade length}}$$

The relationship between pressure in a sphere and

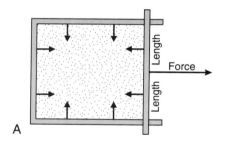

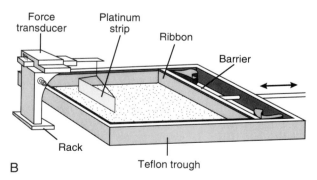

Figure 1–15. Apparatus for measuring surface tension. *A.* Maxwell frame. *B.* Clements frame. (Redrawn from Clements JA, Tierney DF: Alveolar instability associated with altered surface tension. In Fenn WO, Rahn H [eds]: Handbook of Physiology, Section 3, Respiration, vol II, pp. 1565–1583. Washington, DC, American Physiological Society, 1965.)

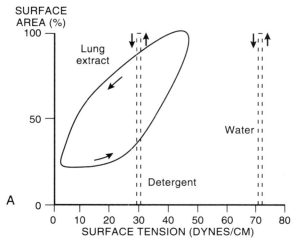
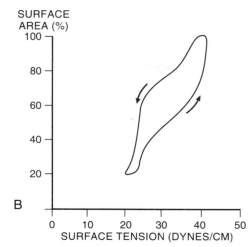

Figure 1–16. *A.* Area–surface tension diagram. Lung extract is pulmonary surfactant (see text). *B.* The area–surface tension diagram of an infant with respiratory distress caused by premature delivery. (*A,* from Comroe JH: Physiology of Respiration, 2nd ed. Chicago, Year Book Medical Publishers, 1975; *B,* courtesy of Dr. John Clements and Dr. William Tooley.)

the tension in the wall is described by the *law of Laplace:*

$$P = \frac{2T}{R}$$

where T is the wall tension (dynes/cm) and R is the radius of the sphere (cm) (see later for the more general form of this equation). The surface tension of water is high (> 70 dynes/cm). Assuming that alveoli are roughly spherical with an average diameter of about ⅓ mm, investigators realized that the lung must contain some mechanism for reducing surface tension. Otherwise, alveoli would be prone to collapse as their volumes changed (see later). In addition, lung inflation would be more difficult because the lung recoil generated by the high surface tension of water would be large. To assess lung surface tension, investigators developed the *Clements frame* (see Figure 1–15B) to study the surface tension properties of fluid washed out of lungs by *alveolar lavage* with saline. This frame uses a blade attached to a force transducer. The blade is lowered into the water surface, and the surface tension is measured directly. As for the Maxwell frame, surface tension equals the force of attraction/length of the blade. Experiments were carried out in which an extract of the lung lavage fluid was added to the frame. Because the extract from the lung was lighter than water it floated on the surface. A special attraction of the Clements frame was the ability to increase or decrease the surface area, thus compressing or decompressing the monolayer of molecules on the surface.

Figure 1–16 shows an area/surface diagram measured with a Clements frame. Note that water has a constant, high surface tension (70 dynes/cm), which is reduced to 30 dynes/cm by commercial detergent. This reduction in surface tension is unaffected by relative area: that is, compressing or decompressing the molecules of this detergent has no effect on its surface tension–reducing properties. This contrasts to the elliptical shape of the area/surface tension curve obtained when lung extract is studied on the surface of the water. There are three remarkable characteristics of this lung extract. First, it reduces surface tension to a maximum of 45 dynes/cm. Second, at low relative areas where the molecules of this lung extract are compressed (corresponding to low lung volumes), this lung extract is an extraordinary detergent; it reduces surface tension to less than 5 dynes/cm. Third, there is hysteresis to the surface tension–reducing properties of this extract that mimics precisely the hysteresis observed in lungs having an air–water interface (see Figure 1–12).

Composition of Human Surfactant

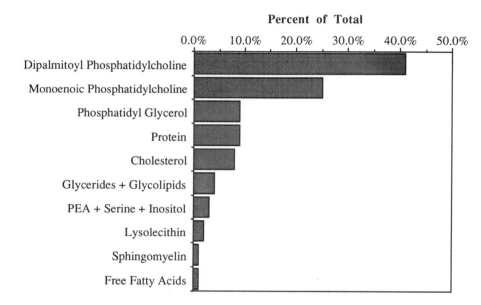

Figure 1-17. The composition of naturally occurring pulmonary surfactant.

This lung extract is called *pulmonary surfactant*. It is a naturally occurring mixture of chemicals, including lipids and protein (Figure 1-17). The predominant ingredient is dipalmitoylphosphatidyl choline (DPPC), which itself has substantial detergent properties. Surfactant is the most effective detergent ever discovered. Recently, synthetic surfactants have become available for treating disease states associated with inadequate surfactant production. For example, premature infants whose lungs have not matured sufficiently to produce normal quantities of surfactant suffer from *respiratory distress of the newborn*. Extract from their lungs fails to reduce surface tension as effectively as shown in Figure 1-16. Because of the resulting high surface tension, many lung units cannot remain open and the gas exchange function of the newborn's lungs is impaired.

By reducing the surface tension in alveoli, surfactant reduces the transmural pressure required to keep alveoli inflated. As a consequence, the pressure difference between alveolar gas and the pressure in the interstitial space surrounding the alveolus is reduced. When alveolar pressure is atmospheric, this causes the interstitial pressure to become less negative. This effect reduces the tendency for fluid to leave the pulmonary capillaries and tends to prevent the development of pulmonary edema (see Chapter 4).

STABILITY OF LUNG UNITS

The pressure term (P) in the Laplace equation (given earlier) can be thought of as the transmural pressure necessary to keep a spherical bubble of liquid inflated to a fixed size. Thus, to maintain an alveolus (assuming spherical geometry) at constant volume, the total tension (T = tissue elastic plus surface tension) in the alveolar wall must be opposed by a transmural distending pressure (P). This is schematized by Figure 1-18, which is a two-dimensional representation of the forces tending to collapse an alveolus and the opposing transmural pressure necessary to hold it at constant volume. This relationship is a consequence of the law of Laplace, which in its most general form is written as

$$P = \frac{2T}{r}$$

where r is the sphere.

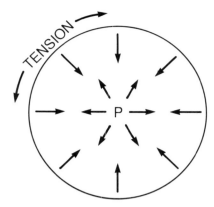

Figure 1–18. Relationship between wall tension (T), which tends to collapse to a lower volume (inward vectors) and the distending pressure (P) necessary to hold the bubble open to a constant volume. This is a two-dimensional rendering of a three-dimensional schema.

Figure 1–19 shows the relationship between volume and transmural pressure (P_{tm}) that would be seen in a spherical alveolus if it contained no surfactant. In the absence of surfactant, the surface tension at the air–liquid interface (T, in the previous equation) would remain constant regardless of the volume of the alveolus. If the alveolus is progressively inflated beginning at a small volume, note that a large increase in transmural pressure is required to produce the first increment in volume (Figure 1–19, $A \rightarrow B$). As the volume increases, the radius of the sphere increases and the transmural pressure required to keep it at any given volume decreases (Figure 1–19, $B \rightarrow C$). Hence, the transmural pressure necessary to keep an alveolus inflated would *decrease* as the transpulmonary pressure (i.e., lung volume) *increases*. Conversely, during lung deflation (Figure 1–19, $B \rightarrow C$) the transpulmonary pressure required to keep smaller alveoli inflated would increase, yet the transpulmonary pressure decreases during exhalation. The relationship shown in Figure 1–19 therefore would cause instability of alveolar inflation and tend to cause alveolar collapse. Addition of surfactant stabilizes the inflation of alveoli because it allows the surface tension (T) to decrease as alveoli become larger. As a result, the transmural pressure required to keep an alveolus inflated increases as lung volume (and transpulmonary pressure) increase and decreases as lung volume decreases. This is shown by the dashed line in Figure 1–19. Thus, surfactant lessens the possibility of alveolar collapse by reducing surface tension to a greater extent in small, as opposed to larger, alveoli.

Another important factor that contributes to alveolar stability is termed *interdependence*. Because alveoli are interconnected by the structural elements of the lung, the collapse of a single alveolus causes stretch and distortion of the surrounding alveoli, which are, in turn, connected to other alveoli, and so on. This mechanical interdependence lessens the ability of alveoli to collapse by providing tethering from the surrounding structures that are ultimately linked to pleural pressure.

REGIONAL COMPLIANCE

The static volume of the entire lung (or a region of the lung) is set by the transmural pressure. Thus far, pleural pressure has been described as a single value throughout the pleural space. If this were true all regions of the lung would be equally distended at any given lung overall transmural pressure. However, a gradient in pleural pressure exists from the top to the bottom of the vertical lung that results (in

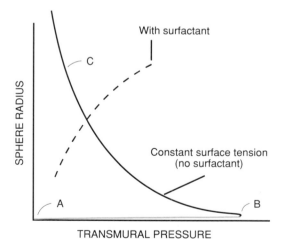

Figure 1–19. Relationship between volume of a bubble and the distending pressure required to maintain that volume. *Solid line.* Bubble has constant surface tension that does not change as a function of volume. *Dashed line.* Surfactant has been added, thereby decreasing surface tension more at small volumes than at large volumes.

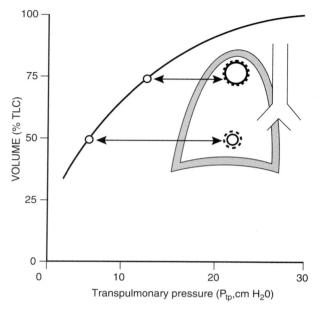

Figure 1–20. Regional differences in lung distention caused by intrathoracic gradient in pleural pressure. This gradient is largely a gravitational effect. (Redrawn from Gibson GJ, Pride NJ: Lung distensibility. Br J Dis Chest 70:143–183, 1976.)

on different parts of the pressure–volume curve, a given change in pleural pressure produces a larger change in volume in alveoli at the bottom than at the top (Figure 1–22). Thus, the effective alveolar ventilation (change in alveolar volume relative to the initial volume) will be greater in alveoli near the base than in the apex of the upright lung. By analogy, when the Slinky spring is stretched the coils

part) from the effects of gravity. Consequently, the pleural pressure is more negative near the top of the lung than at the bottom. Thus, when alveolar pressure is the same as atmospheric pressure in all alveoli (e.g., at FRC with the glottis open) the lung transmural pressure is greater at the top of the lung than at the bottom. For example, at FRC, P_{pl} is about -10 cm H_2O at the apex of the vertical lung and about -2.5 cm H_2O at the base.

Figure 1–20 shows how this effect causes alveoli near the top of the lung to assume a larger volume at FRC than alveoli near the bottom — they lie at different points along the pressure–volume relationship. This situation is analogous to a metal Slinky Toy spring, held vertically (Figure 1–21). When the spring is allowed to hang freely, the weight of the spring stretches the coils farther apart near the top than at the bottom (alveolar volumne at FRC is smaller at the base than apex).

As inspiration occurs, the pleural pressure changes by equal amounts at the top and the bottom of the lung. Accordingly, the *change* in transpulmonary pressure is identical at the top and bottom of the lung. However, because the top and bottom are

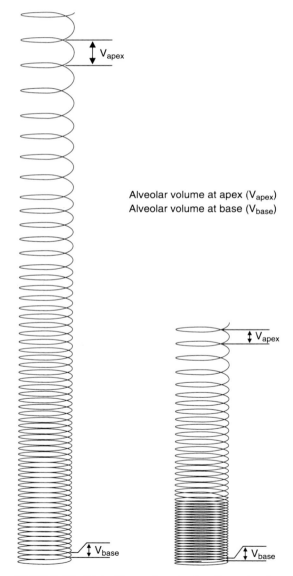

Figure 1–21. Slinky Toy analogy to describe regional differences in lung volume and ventilation.

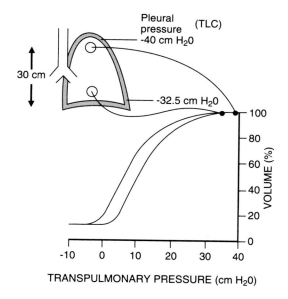

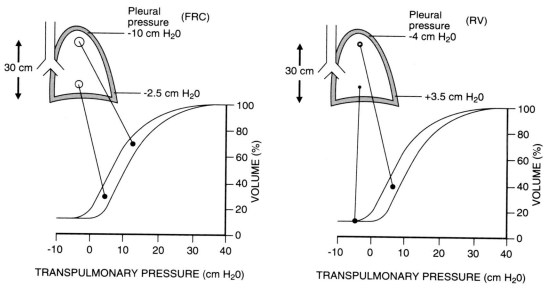

Figure 1–22. Effect of gradient in pleural pressure on regional ventilation during inspiration at various lung volumes (see text for discussion).

near the bottom separate more, relative to their initial spacing, than the coils near the top. Thus, the change in spacing divided by the initial spacing of the coils is large for the bottom of the spring but relatively small for coils near the top. This effect gives rise to *regional differences in ventilation*, which influence the gas exchange function of the lung (see Chapter 7). Note that if a subject lies down, the gradient in pleural pressure switches to the antero-posterior direction.

Chapter 2

Lung Mechanics: Dynamics

Air is a fluid, and the principles that govern its movement in and out of the lung are those of *fluid dynamics*. Dynamics is that aspect of mechanics that studies physical systems in motion. By application of Newton's law of motion, the mechanisms that affect the flow of air into and out of the lung in health and in diseases are defined.

APPLICATIONS OF FLUID MECHANICS

Flow Regimens in Airways

Fluid flow will occur along a rigid tube when a hydrostatic pressure difference exists between one end of the tube and the other. In airways, gas flow will occur when a pressure difference exists between one point along the airway and another, as long as the airway is open and a free path for gas flow

exists. When a fluid flows along a tube, the *average velocity* (speed, in cm/sec) can be calculated by dividing the overall flow rate (ml/sec) by the cross-sectional area of the tube (cm²).

Fluid movement can be *laminar* or *turbulent* or may have characteristics intermediate between these two extremes (Figure 2-1). In laminar or stream-lined flow, the fluid traveling at the center of the tube moves most rapidly, while the fluid in direct contact with the tube wall remains stationary. If water flows down a pipe under laminar conditions, a small stream of ink injected at the center of the pipe will tend to stay at the center of the flow stream as it travels down the tube. Another stream of ink injected between the center of the pipe and the wall will also travel in a straight line but will move down the pipe more slowly. One way to imagine this is to think of the fluid as if it were composed of a series of concentric tubes sliding past

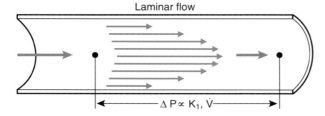

Laminar flow

$$\Delta P \propto K_1, \dot{V}$$

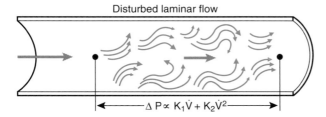

Disturbed laminar flow

$$\Delta P \propto K_1 \dot{V} + K_2 \dot{V}^2$$

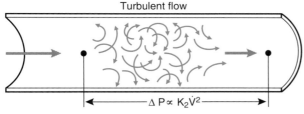

Turbulent flow

$$\Delta P \propto K_2 \dot{V}^2$$

Figure 2–1. Laminar, disturbed, and turbulent flow conditions. All flow travels parallel to the axis of the tube under laminar flow conditions. Fluid at the center of the tube moves at a higher velocity than flow near the tube boundary. Eddies and vortices disrupt the flow pattern in turbulent flow states. Although net movement of fluid occurs along the tube, turbulent eddies generate flows perpendicular to the tube axis. This process consumes energy, causing a steeper drop in pressure along the tube than in laminar flow regimens. In disturbed laminar flow, characteristics of both laminar and turbulent flow are present.

each other, much like a radio aerial being pulled out. Because the fluid velocity decreases with the square of the radial distance away from the center of the tube, laminar flow is said to have a *parabolic* velocity profile. In laminar flow regimens, the *average* fluid velocity in the tube is half of the *peak* velocity seen at the center of the tube. Laminar flow does not begin at the entrance of the pipe, since the fluid must travel some distance down the pipe for laminar flow conditions to become fully established.

In *marginally laminar* or *disturbed* flow, characteristics of both laminar and turbulent flow can be seen. Flow is generally laminar, but eddies are generated at sites where the tube narrows or branches

or changes dimensions or where irregularities in the tube surface are encountered. This flow regimen is similar to the pattern of eddies seen as water vapor rises above a cup of hot tea.

In *fully turbulent* flow, fluid movement occurs both in *radial* (i.e., perpendicular to the axis of the tube) and *axial* directions. Although fluid in contact with the tube wall still remains stationary, the velocity profile across the tube is much more blunt than the parabolic profile seen in laminar flow; there is less variation in fluid velocity as a function of radial position in the tube. Because fluid moving in a radial direction can impact on the tube wall, noise is often generated in turbulent flow states. Since energy is consumed in the process of generating the eddies and chaotic fluid movement, a higher driving pressure is required to support a given flow rate under turbulent as opposed to laminar flow conditions, other factors remaining the same.

Under laminar flow conditions, the pressure difference between two points along a tube is directly proportional to the flow rate:

$$\Delta P = k_1 \cdot \dot{V}$$

where ΔP is the pressure difference (cm H_2O), k_1 is a resistive constant for the system (cm $H_2O \cdot sec/ml$) and $\dot{V}$ is flow rate (ml/sec). (Note that the dot above the $\dot{V}$ signifies *change in volume with respect to time*, i.e., flow rate). Stated alternatively, the driving pressure (ΔP) along a tube must be doubled to double the flow rate during laminar flow. In turbulent flow conditions, the pressure difference between two points along the tube increases with the square of the flow rate. Thus, doubling the flow under turbulent conditions requires more than a doubling of the driving pressure, since some of the fluid moves perpendicular to the axis of the tube. The relationship between driving pressure and flow for a turbulent system can be approximated by:

$$\Delta P \approx k_2 \cdot \dot{V}^2$$

where ΔP is the pressure difference, k_2 is a constant for the system, and $\dot{V}$ is flow. Thus, there is a linear relationship between pressure and flow under laminar conditions and a nonlinear relationship under turbulent conditions. Figure 2–2 shows this relationship graphically. During tidal breathing, fluid flow is highly turbulent in the trachea, is less turbu-

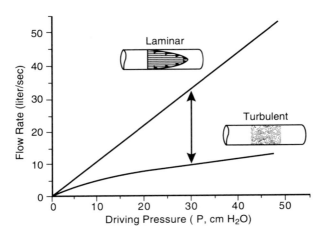

Figure 2–2. Relationship between driving pressure and flow through a pipe under laminar and turbulent flow conditions. During laminar flow, an increase in the driving pressure produces a proportionate increase in flow rate. In turbulent flow states, the same increase in pressure augments flow to a lesser degree, since some of the increase in driving pressure moves fluid in a direction perpendicular to the tube axis.

lent in smaller bronchi, and finally becomes laminar-like in the small peripheral airways. Therefore, the total pressure drop that occurs between alveoli and the mouth during inhalation includes some contribution from laminar-like flow plus some contribution from turbulent flow regimens. This can be approximated using the following relationship:

$$\Delta P \approx k_1 \cdot \dot{V} + k_2 \cdot \dot{V}^2$$

This equation states that the total pressure difference between an alveolus and the mouth (ΔP) is the sum of the pressure drop encountered in laminar flow regions (small airways) and in turbulent flow regions (larger airways).

Reynolds Number and Turbulent Flow

It is possible to predict whether flow in a system will tend to be laminar or turbulent by calculating the *Reynolds number* (Re).

$$Re = \frac{(D \cdot u \cdot \rho)}{\eta}$$

where ρ is the density of the fluid (g/ml), D is the diameter of the tube or airway (cm), u is the average velocity (cm/sec), and η is the viscosity of the fluid (g/[sec · cm]). Reynolds number is a dimensionless value because it expresses the ratio of two dimensionally equivalent terms (kinematic/viscous). For any fluid, flow generally tends to be turbulent when Re is greater than 2000 and laminar when Re is less than 2000, although this is only an approximation.

During normal tidal breathing, gas flows of 1 liter/sec are common at the mouth. In an adult trachea with a diameter of 3 cm, this will produce tracheal gas velocities of about 150 cm/sec. Since air has a density of about 0.0012 g/ml and a viscosity of 1.83×10^{-4} g/(sec · cm), the calculated Reynolds number in a trachea with diameter of 3 cm (more than 2000) indicates that flow in the trachea is highly turbulent even during quiet breathing. The open glottis and the vocal cords introduce mechanical obstructions that further promote the tendency to develop turbulence. However, since the total cross-sectional area of the airways expands enormously from the central to the peripheral regions of the lung, gas velocities decrease significantly in the more distal (i.e., toward the alveoli) airways. This greatly lessens the tendency for flow to be turbulent in the lung periphery, even during maximal ventilation. The increase in total cross-sectional area of the airways toward the lung periphery has been compared with the shape of a thumbtack (Figure 2–3). Because the individual airways decrease in diameter toward the lung periphery, the tendency for turbulent flow to occur is even further reduced. Therefore, the flow regimens in the lung are highly turbulent in the larger airways but never turbulent in the small distal airways.

RESISTANCE TO AIRFLOW

Pressure–Flow Relationships in Airways

When flow in a tube is laminar, there is a linear relationship between driving pressure and flow (see Figure 2–2). Flow is set both by the driving pressure applied and the *resistance* to flow in the system. Under laminar conditions:

$$\dot{V} = \frac{\Delta P}{R}$$

where $\dot{V}$ is flow, ΔP is driving pressure from one end of the system to other, and R is resistance over the same distance. As driving pressure increases, flow increases proportionally as long as resistance in the system remains constant. In other words, the resistance to flow is defined as the pressure difference required to maintain a given flow rate through a system.

Poiseuille's law defines the relationship between flow and pressure in a tube with fixed dimensions, under *laminar* flow conditions:

$$\dot{V} = \frac{(\Delta P \cdot \pi \cdot r^4)}{(8 \cdot \eta \cdot L)}$$

where ΔP is the pressure drop along a tube, $\dot{V}$ is the flow rate, η is the fluid viscosity, L is the length of the tube, and r is the tube radius. From the above equation, the resistance term is represented by the following equation:

$$Resistance = \frac{8 \cdot \eta \cdot L}{\pi \cdot r^4}$$

Note that for any given fluid, the pressure difference required to drive a given flow rate is directly proportional to the length of the tube but is inversely proportional to the fourth power of the radius of the tube. Thus for a given driving pressure difference, doubling the length of the tube will halve the flow rate, whereas halving the tube diameter will decrease the flow 16 times under laminar flow conditions. Stated differently, the resistance is inversely proportional to the radius raised to the fourth power but directly proportional to the length of the tube and the viscosity of the fluid. Clearly, the tube radius is the dominant factor in determining the resistance to flow.

Airflow Velocity

Flow in a tube possesses energy in two different forms. *Kinetic energy* is that part of the total energy associated with bulk movement of the fluid and is related to the density of the fluid (ρ, in g/ml) and the square of the average velocity (u^2):

$$Kinetic\ energy = \tfrac{1}{2}\,\rho u^2$$

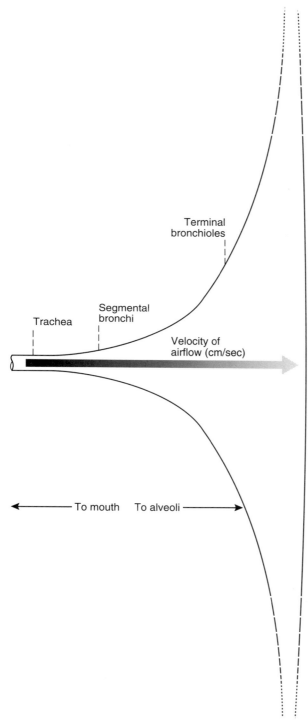

Figure 2-3. Total airway cross-sectional area as a function of distance into the lung. Although the diameters of individual airways become smaller toward the lung periphery, the number of airways increases dramatically. Accordingly, the total airway cross-sectional area increases markedly toward the alveoli and gas velocities decrease.

The second form of energy is *potential energy,* and in airways the hydrostatic pressure is the major component of this. The *total energy* of the fluid flow is the sum of the potential and kinetic energy components. As fluid travels along a pipe, frictional resistance decreases the total energy of the flow. This is seen as a decrease in the pressure component of the total energy (i.e., the hydrostatic pressure decreases along the tube, reflecting frictional loss of pressure energy). If the velocity of the flow changes along the tube, then a greater proportion of the total energy is converted from potential (pressure) to kinetic energy. This concept is demonstrated in Figure 2–4, which illustrates the events that occur as a fluid flows along a tube whose diameter narrows. In this figure, a gas flow of 1 liter/sec travels down a tube with a diameter of 3 cm and a cross-sectional area of 7.06 cm². At a point along the tube, the diameter tapers to 2.1 cm, so that the area (3.53 cm²) is half of the original area. Since the average velocity (cm/sec) of gas in the tube is calculated by dividing the flow rate (cm³/sec) by the area of the tube (cm²), the fluid must accelerate from 140 cm/sec to 280 cm/sec as it enters the narrow section. The energy used to accelerate the fluid comes from the potential (pressure) energy. Hence, the hydrostatic pressure falls within the narrow portion of the tube because the kinetic energy has increased at the expense of the pressure energy component. At the end of the narrow segment the fluid decelerates and the veloc-

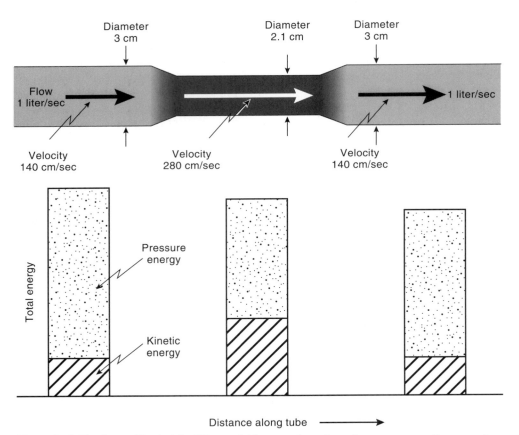

Figure 2–4. The Bernoulli principle. When a fluid moves through a tube at a constant flow rate, the total energy of the fluid (potential energy + kinetic energy) decreases because frictional losses convert some of the energy into heat. Increases in fluid velocity occur where the tube narrows, causing an increase in the kinetic energy component (½ ρu^2) at the expense of potential energy (pressure decreases). When the tube widens again, the fluid decelerates and kinetic energy is converted into pressure energy.

ity of flow decreases. The corresponding loss in kinetic energy is converted back to pressure energy, so the hydrostatic pressure rises. As all of this occurs, there is still a progressive loss in the total energy of the fluid along the tube, because resistive losses cause the conversion of some of the energy into heat. At the exit of the tube, the kinetic energy component is the same as was present at the start of the tube, because the velocities are the same. However, the total energy is reduced because the pressure component is smaller. The key point to remember is that when velocity speeds up because a tube narrows, the hydrostatic pressure decreases as a result. This phenomenon is referred to as the *Bernoulli effect.* Note from Figure 2–2 that during an exhalation, gas velocity must increase dramatically as flow travels toward the trachea, because the total airway area decreases. This causes the hydrostatic pressure to fall within the airways, an effect that becomes very important during forceful exhalations (discussed later).

The Respiratory Cycle

Exchange of oxygen and carbon dioxide between alveolar gas and pulmonary capillary blood occurs as these gases move passively (i.e., *diffuse*) from regions of higher *partial pressure* to regions of lower partial pressure. To maintain the partial pressure differences driving diffusion in the alveoli, the heart must continually pump blood through the pulmonary circulation and the respiratory system must continually deliver fresh gas to the alveoli. Moreover, blood flow and alveolar ventilation must be adjusted to accommodate a wide range of metabolic rates, ranging from resting states to maximal exercise.

The *minute ventilation* is the volume of gas breathed per minute. This involves the bulk (convective) movement of air into and out of the lungs. Ventilation is normally achieved by periodic breathing or *tidal ventilation.* During inhalation, the diaphragm and the inspiratory muscles of the chest wall shorten, causing the diaphragm to move downward and the chest wall to move upward and outward. This process lowers the hydrostatic pressure in the pleural space by expanding the chest volume. Since the lungs are not rigid structures, the decrease in pleural pressure is transmitted across

the visceral pleural surface into the lungs, causing alveolar hydrostatic pressure to fall. When alveolar pressure becomes less than ambient pressure, gas flows into the lungs (assuming that the glottis and airways are open) until the alveolar hydrostatic pressure rises to the ambient pressure. At this point (end-inspiration), the hydrostatic pressure difference between alveolar gas and ambient air is zero, so inspiratory flow ceases. Note also that at end-inspiration the force generated by the contracting inspiratory muscles equals the elastic force generated by the lungs and chest wall. At the beginning of exhalation, the diaphragm and other inspiratory muscles relax. This causes the hydrostatic pressure in the pleural space to increase, as the elastic (potential) energy stored in the lung and chest wall and abdomen begin to compress the thoracic contents. Once again, the change in pleural hydrostatic pressure is transmitted across the visceral pleura to alveolar gas, causing its pressure to rise above the ambient pressure. If the airway remains open, gas flows out of the lung until alveolar pressure decreases to equal ambient atmospheric pressure.

Figure 2–5 details this sequence of events that occur during a single breath, assuming that the airway and glottis remain open throughout. First, consider the situation existing at the instant before the breath begins (point A in Figure 2–5). At this point, inspiratory and expiratory muscles are relaxed, so the lung is at end-expiratory volume (i.e., functional residual capacity [FRC]). At that point, airflow is absent because alveolar pressure is equal to ambient atmospheric pressure (i.e., no pressure gradient between alveoli and atmospheric exists). Pleural pressure is -7.5 cm H_2O at point A, so *transpulmonary pressure* (P_{tp}) (i.e., the transmural pressure for the lung, defined as alveolar $[P_{alv}]$ minus pleural pressure $[P_{pl}]$) is:

$$P_{tp} = P_{alv} - P_{pl} = 0 - (-7.5)$$

$$= +7.5 \text{ cm } H_2O.$$

Transmural pressure for the chest wall at point A would then be:

$$P_{trans-chest\ wall} = P_{pl} - P_{atmospheric}$$

$$= (-7.5) - 0 = -7.5 \text{ cm } H_2O.$$

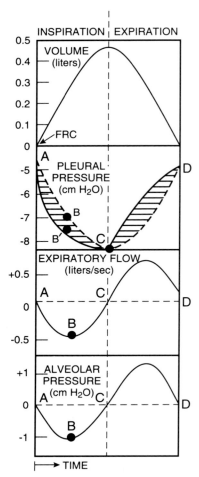

Figure 2–5. Changes in pleural and alveolar pressures during a tidal breath. Note that whenever lung volume is not changing with time, lung volume is determined by transpulmonary pressure. See text for further explanation. (Adapted and redrawn from West JB: Respiratory Physiology: The Essentials, 4th ed. © 1985, the Williams & Wilkins, Co., Baltimore.)

The positive transmural pressure for the lung indicates that the lung is being held open at FRC by a positive distending pressure. By contrast, the negative resting transmural pressure for the chest wall at FRC indicates that the chest wall is being pulled in by a negative distending pressure. The negative pleural pressure at FRC reflects a balance between this tendency for the lung to collapse toward a smaller volume and the tendency for the chest wall to spring out to a larger volume. Stated differently, FRC is defined as the lung volume at which

the negative transmural pressure for the relaxed chest wall (-7.5 cm H_2O) matches the positive transmural pressure for the lung ($+7.5$ cm H_2O) (see Chapter 1). At these matching transmural pressures, both the lung and the relaxed chest wall have the same volume (an anatomical necessity).

At the start of inhalation, the diaphragm and other inspiratory muscles shorten, causing chest volume to expand and pleural pressure to decrease. The decrease in pleural pressure is transmitted through the lung visceral pleura to the alveolar space, causing alveolar pressure to decrease. Approximately halfway through inspiration (point B in Figure 2–5) the inspiratory flow rate is maximal because alveolar pressure is maximally negative. At end-inspiration (point C), alveolar pressure again rises to ambient pressure and so inspiratory flow ceases. At that instant, pleural pressure is about -11 cm H_2O, so transmural pressures are:

$$P_{tp} = P_{alv} - P_{pl} = 0 - (-11)$$
$$= +11 \text{ cm } H_2O.$$

This higher static transpulmonary pressure is associated with a lung volume that is about 500 ml above FRC. Transmural pressure for the chest wall at point A would then be:

$$P_{trans-chest \ wall} = P_{pl} - P_{atmospheric}$$
$$= (-11) - 0 = -11 \text{ cm } H_2O.$$

Note that the transmural pressure for the chest wall is more negative, yet the thoracic volume is larger! This occurs because the respiratory muscles are contracting, thereby dramatically altering the mechanical properties of the chest wall relative to its relaxed (i.e., passive) pressure–volume relationship.

During exhalation, the cycle is reversed and lung volume returns from end-inspiration to FRC. This is associated with a return of pleural pressure from -11 cm H_2O to -7.5 cm H_2O. At point D, the conditions of physiological equilibrium at FRC again are established as at point A and the cycle is completed.

Lung Resistance

The pleural pressure curve AB'C (see Figure 2–5) represents the change in pleural pressure seen during tidal breathing. The dashed line ABC represents the pleural pressure curve that *would have been required* to inflate the same lung very slowly; that is, it reflects the pressure–volume relationship of the lung obtained under quasi-static conditions. Note that during a normal inspiration, pleural pressure transiently becomes more negative (AB'C) than it would during a very slow inflation (ABC). Likewise, during exhalation pleural pressure transiently rises above the level that would occur during a very slow exhalation.

The difference between curve ABC and curve AB'C represents the additional pressure necessary to overcome the resistance encountered while *changing* lung volume. This impedance to changing lung volume is termed *lung resistance*. Note that when lung volume is not changing with time (i.e., at end-inspiration or end-expiration), the transpulmonary pressure is identical to what would occur during a static lung inflation to that volume. While lung volume is changing, the additional pleural pressure required to overcome lung resistance depends on how fast the lung volume is changing. Thus, to decrease lung volume rapidly, a larger increment in pleural pressure is required than would be needed to decrease lung volume slowly. Two factors contribute to this lung resistance. Part of the lung resistance arises from the pressure drop created by gas flow in the airways, as gas enters or leaves the lung *(airways resistance)*. One component of the airways resistance is due to *frictional resistance* to airflow. Another part is due to the *acceleration* (or deceleration) of gas to a higher (or lower) velocity as it moves away from (or toward) the lung periphery as a result of the changing total cross-sectional area (see Figure 2–2). The second factor contributing to lung resistance reflects the viscous impedance encountered in changing lung volume, separate and apart from the gas flow resistance *(viscous contribution)*.

This situation is somewhat analogous to inflating and deflating an old fireplace bellows equipped with a spring (Figure 2–6). Inflating the bellows

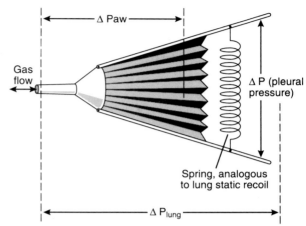

Figure 2–6. By analogy, respiratory system resistance is similar to the resistance encountered in operating a fireplace bellows (with the spring detached). Part of the resistance encountered is due to the work of driving flow through airways that narrow in total area from the alveolus toward the mouth (airways resistance). Another component relates to the resistance in moving the bellows itself, as would be encountered if operated in a vacuum (tissue viscous resistance). The spring represents the force that would be required to operate the bellows very slowly (static lung recoil).

very slowly requires an increasing force to overcome the elastic pull of the spring (static lung recoil). Inflating the bellows more rapidly *requires an additional force at any given volume,* owing to the bellow's resistance to changing volume (analogous to lung resistance). Because of this resistance, the more rapidly the bellows is inflated the greater the force required. Part of the overall resistance arises from the intrinsic resistance of the bellows itself. This is the resistance to movement offered by the moving parts of the bellows, analogous to the viscous component of lung resistance. In effect, this is the resistance to movement that would be encountered if the spring were removed and the bellows was operated in a vacuum environment. Most of the bellow's resistance to movement is due to the impedance to airflow through the spout (airways resistance). Thus, narrowing the diameter of the spout will increase the force needed to inflate the bellows at a given rate (increased frictional and accelerative contributions). By analogy, airways resistance is the resistance encountered if the bellows were operated with the spring removed and the viscous component subtracted.

The *viscous* component of lung resistance (analo-

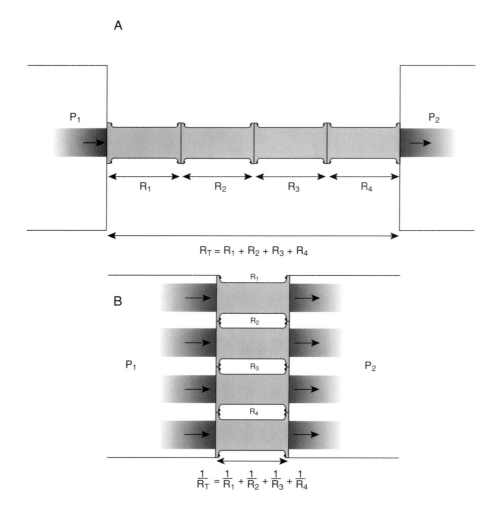

Figure 2-7. Resistance to fluid flow through four pipe segments, arranged sequentially in series *(A)* or in parallel (B). The total resistance (R_T) is the sum of individual resistances when arranged in series. When arranged in parallel, the total resistance is less than for any single segment because multiple separate pathways exist.

gous to the impedance offered by the moving parts of the bellows) varies with lung volume and can also be influenced by other factors. Sometimes called *tissue viscous resistance* or *lung viscance*, this component of lung resistance is generally small during normal tidal breathing. Airways resistance is the major component of lung resistance in the normal lung.

Lung resistance at a given lung volume can be measured during tidal breathing by subtracting the static lung transpulmonary pressure contribution from the total pressure difference between pleural pressure and the pressure at the airway opening. [In the fireplace bellows analogy, this is similar to measuring the resistance to operating the bellows while

the spring is removed.] In practice, a balloon catheter is advanced down the esophagus to measure pleural pressure, as was used for determination of the static pressure–volume relationship described in Chapter 1. Because lung resistance decreases as lung volume increases, repeated measurements of lung resistance will differ unless the measurements are all made at the same lung volume. For this reason, repeated measurements are generally made at the same point in the ventilatory cycle (i.e., at mid-inspiration or mid-expiration). Referring to Figure 2–5, the pleural pressure at mid-inspiration (point B) is -7.5 cm H_2O. At that lung volume, the static pleural pressure would be -7.0 cm H_2O (point B′). Thus, the magnitude of the pleural pressure is 0.5

cm H_2O greater than would be seen with a static inflation at that lung volume. At point B, flow is 0.5 liter/sec. Recall that resistance is defined as a pressure difference divided by flow. The pressure difference created by the flow is therefore 0.5 cm H_2O minus the pressure at the airway opening (0 cm H_2O):

$$R = \frac{\Delta P}{\Delta \dot{V}}$$

$$R_L = \frac{0.5 \text{ cm } H_2O}{0.5 \text{ liter/sec}}$$

$$R_L = 1.0 \; \frac{\text{cm } H_2O}{\text{liter/sec}}$$

where R_L is the symbol for lung resistance (flow + viscous components) and cm H_2O/(liter/sec) is the unit of lung resistance. This lung resistance (1.0 cm H_2O/[liter/sec]) is typical of that which occurs in a normal adult human during inspiration.

Distribution of Lung Resistance

When laminar flow occurs through a branched system of tubes, the overall resistance across the system depends on the individual resistances in each pipe and the manner in which the pipes are connected. Figure 2–7 shows an arrangement of four pipe segments, each with a flow resistance of 1 torr/(liter/sec). When connected in series, the resistance of the network equals the sum of the individual resistances:

$$R_{Total} = R_1 + R_2 + R_3 + R_4$$

$$R_{Total} = 1 + 1 + 1 + 1 = 4$$

However, if the pipes are arranged in parallel (Figure 2–7B) the total resistance across the network will be less than the resistance of any single pipe. In this example, four simultaneous pathways exist, so the total resistance is only one-fourth of the resistance of any single segment. In general, the total resistance (R_{Total}) across a group of resistances arranged in parallel can be calculated using the relationship

$$\frac{1}{R_T} = \frac{1}{R_1} + \frac{1}{R_2} + \frac{1}{R_3} + \; . \; . \; .$$

As airways travel from the trachea toward the alveoli, they branch successively into daughter airways. At each branch point, the daughter airways are described as belonging to the next *generation*. In general, airways of similar generation number tend to be about the same diameter. In moving from the trachea to the periphery of the lung the airways increase in number as they branch, but the individual bronchi become progressively smaller in diameter. The smaller diameter tends to increase the resistance offered by each bronchus, but the large increase in the number of parallel pathways tends to reduce the overall resistance encountered at each generation of branching. This can be described as a network of resistances, as shown in Figure 2–8. The collective resistance contributed by each generation reflects a balance between the number of airways in parallel and the radius of each. Figure 2–9 shows the relative resistances encountered at each airway generation. If the trachea is considered as generation 0, resistance increases slightly for the first few generations, reaching a peak near generations 3 to 6 (corresponding to segmental bronchi). Beyond this level, the increase in the number of parallel airways outweighs the decrease in diameter of each bronchus, causing the resistance at further generations to decrease progressively. At the level of the terminal bronchioles (generation 16), the airways resistance is a small fraction of the resistance in the segmental bronchi. During normal breathing, approximately 80% of the resistance to airflow at FRC is in airways whose diameters exceed 2 mm.

Measurement of Airways Resistance

By measuring pleural pressure and airflow simultaneously, lung resistance can be determined during tidal breathing if the static volume–pressure relationship of the lung is known. Theoretically, airways resistance could be calculated by subtracting the viscous component from the measured lung resistance. However, the viscous component of lung resistance is difficult to measure directly, so this approach is not practical. Moreover, lung resistance itself is difficult to measure in the clinical setting because it requires the placement of a balloon-tipped catheter at the correct position in the esophagus.

The direct measurement of airways resistance re-

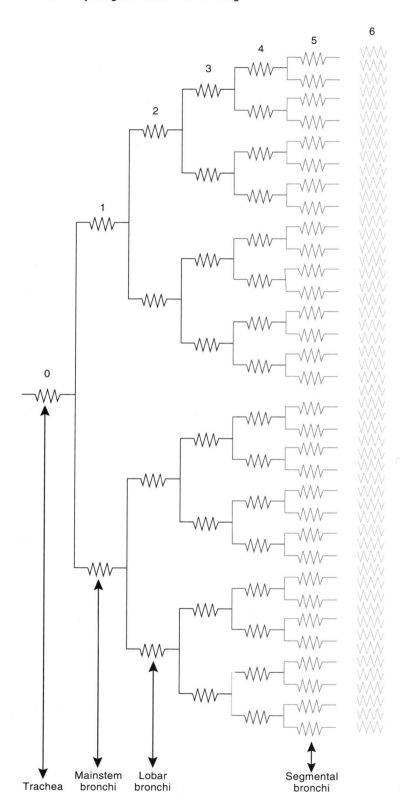

Figure 2-8. Airway resistance as a function of airway generation. The resistance contribution of any given airway generation (i.e., all the airways of that generation taken collectively) reflects a balance between the number of airways of that generation (arranged in parallel) and the individual resistance of each. Most of the overall airway resistance normally resides in generations 0 through 8. The contribution of resistance contributed by higher generations is relatively less because the number of smaller airways is large relative to their individual resistances.

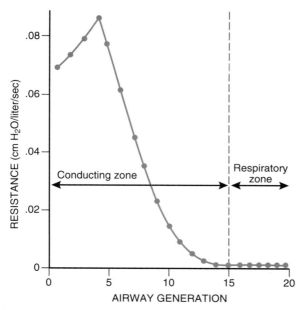

Figure 2-9. Airways resistance as a function of airway generation. In the normal lung, most of the resistance to airflow occurs in the first eight airway generations. (Redrawn from Pedley TJ et al: The prediction of pressure drop and variation of resistance within the human bronchial airways. Respir Physiol 9:387, 1970.)

quires that the alveolar-minus-mouth pressure difference be measured simultaneously with gas flow rate during a breath. This can be accomplished using a *body plethysmograph,* shown in Figure 2-10.

A subject fitted with a nose clip is seated inside a sealed body plethysmograph. The subject breathes air through a mouthpiece, equipped with an electrically operated occlusive shutter (normally open). A flow transducer attached to the mouthpiece measures the airflow rate as the subject breathes in and out. At the end of a passive exhalation (i.e., at FRC) the technologist closes the shutter to prevent airflow and asks the subject to pant rapidly against the closed shutter (see Figure 2-10A). When the shutter is closed, neither inspiration nor expiration can occur, so the pressure in the mouth is the same as alveolar pressure. This mouth pressure (P_M) is measured using a pressure transducer, as is the pressure in the box (P_B). When P_M is plotted as a function of P_B, a straight line is obtained with a slope of $\Delta P_M/\Delta P_B$. The airway shutter is then opened (see Figure 2-10B) and the subject is again asked to pant at FRC. During this procedure, the instantaneous flow

at the mouth ($\dot{V}_M$) is measured, along with the pressure in the box (P_B). When $\dot{V}_M$ is plotted as a function of P_B, another straight line is obtained with a slope $\Delta\dot{V}_M/\Delta P_B$. From the closed shutter maneuver, the alveolar pressure corresponding to a given box pressure is known. Applying this to the open shutter, panting allows the alveolar pressure to be calculated from the measured box pressure. This calculation is made by dividing the slope of the $\Delta P_M/\Delta P_B$ line by the slope of the $\Delta\dot{V}_M/\Delta P_B$ line:

$$\frac{(\Delta P_M/\Delta P_B)}{(\Delta\dot{V}_M/\Delta P_B)} = \frac{\Delta P_M}{\Delta\dot{V}_M} = Raw$$

This yields a ratio of alveolar pressure to flow. Since the pressure at the mouth remains atmospheric during the open-shutter panting maneuver, this ratio is equal to the airways resistance, Raw.

The measurement of airways resistance with the body plethysmograph is relatively simple and can be combined with the measurement of FRC (see Chapter 1). Since panting with the shutter open only changes lung volume by about 50 ml, this measurement of Raw effectively avoids the changes in airway resistance that occur when lung volume changes (see later). This technique to assess Raw has become the standard for measuring resistance to airflow in clinical assessments of lung volume.

Airways Resistance and Lung Volume

Resistance to airflow changes markedly at different lung volumes. For this reason, measurements of lung resistance or airways resistance should always be made at a known lung volume. Since FRC is a volume that is easily reproducible, and since it is the volume at which persons normally breathe, measurements of resistance are usually made at FRC or some increment above FRC. Figure 2-11 shows how lung resistance varies as a function of lung volume in normal subjects. Lung resistance is highest at low lung volumes and lowest at high lung volumes. Two factors contribute to this volume dependence.

At higher lung volumes, the alveoli are more distended and the elastic tension in the alveolar walls is higher. Bronchi coursing through the lung parenchyma are surrounded by and attached to alveoli and are pulled open by the elastic tension in the

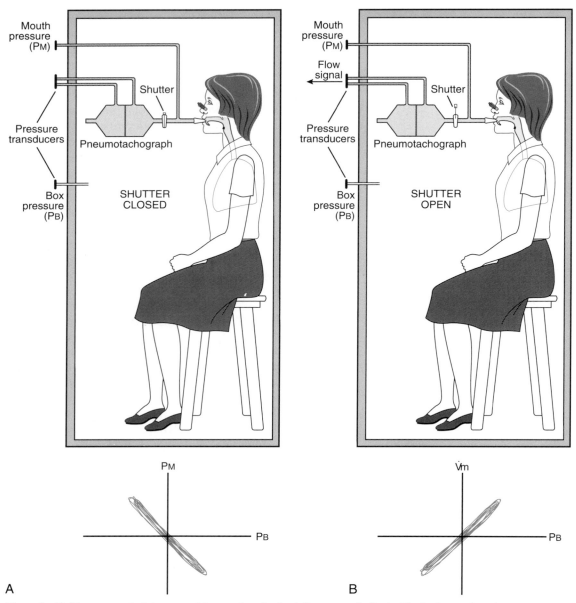

Figure 2–10. Measurement of airways resistance using a body plethysmograph. See text for further explanation.

alveolar walls. Because the bronchi have relatively distensible walls, their caliber (and therefore their resistance) is influenced to a great extent by this mechanical *tethering* effect. At low lung volumes approaching residual volume, tension in alveolar walls is less, so the tethering of the bronchi is reduced and airway resistance is increased. Moreover, some airways begin to close at these low lung vol-

umes *(closing volume)*, further increasing the overall resistance to airflow.

The second factor contributing to the change in lung resistance at different lung volumes arises from changes in autonomic *parasympathetic nervous system* tone with lung volume. During inspiration, specialized neural mechanoreceptors *(stretch receptors)* within the smooth muscle layers in airway

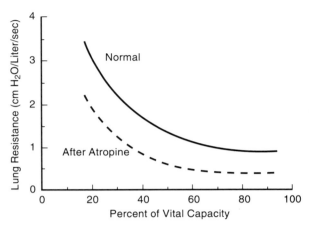

Figure 2-11. Lung resistance as a function of lung inflation. Airways resistance decreases as lung volume increases. At lung volumes above functional residual capacity the airways resistance decreases because (1) increased tension in alveolar septal walls is transmitted to adjacent airways, increasing their diameter, and (2) distention of airway stretch receptors elicits a reflex decrease in parasympathetic nervous system tone, causing a decrease in airway smooth muscle tension. Dashed line shows the effect of atropine (inhibiting parasympathetic effects) on airways resistance. (Redrawn from Vincent NJ, et al: J Appl Physiol 29:236-243, 1970.)

walls detect the increase in lung volume. Mechanical stretch of these receptors at higher lung volumes causes their neural rate of firing to increase. This afferent information is transmitted to the autonomic centers in the brain stem by way of the vagus nerve, and it elicits a reflex decrease in efferent parasympathetic tone (Chapter 12). Decreases in parasympathetic neural tone tend to reduce the active constriction of airway smooth muscle cells *(bronchomotor tone),* thereby reducing airways resistance by increasing airway diameter. Conversely, during exhalation lung volume decreases and parasympathetic tone increases, causing a greater constriction of airway smooth muscle and a greater airflow resistance. Atropine, a drug that blocks the effects of the parasympathetic nervous system by inhibiting postganglionic parasympathetic receptors, diminishes the effects of lung volume on lung resistance (see Figure 2-11). However, atropine does not affect the change in resistance caused by the mechanical tethering of the airways.

DETERMINANTS OF MAXIMUM AIRFLOW

The respiratory system exhibits an enormous reserve capacity, relative to the demands faced at rest.

For example, at rest, an adult human normally breathes 7 to 10 liters of air per minute (the *minute ventilation*). However, during strenuous exercise the minute ventilation can exceed 100 liters/min. In healthy young subjects asked to breathe as hard as possible for 15 seconds, a *maximal voluntary ventilation* (or *ventilation capacity*) of 200 liters/min may be achieved. This ability to augment greatly ventilation contributes to the wide physiological range of metabolic rates that a healthy subject can achieve. Because this reserve capacity of the respiratory system is so large, lung diseases can often progress to advanced stages without infringing on the ability of the respiratory system to meet resting needs. To detect advancing lung disease, several clinical pulmonary function measurements attempt to stress the capacity of the respiratory system. One such measurement is the forced exhalation test.

Flow During Maximal Expiration

Recall from Chapter 1 that a spirogram can be used to record changes in lung volume during quiet breathing, as well as during submaximal or maximal inspirations or expirations. The spirogram records changes in volume (ΔV, in liters, on the y-axis) as a function of time (Δt, in seconds, on the x-axis). Note that the slope of any line on a spirogram has units of $\Delta V / \Delta t$ (in liters/sec), which is equivalent to flow rate. Typically, the subject is asked to inhale to total

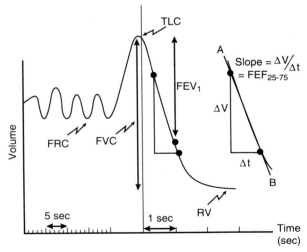

Figure 2-12. Tracing from a spirometer during measurement of a forced expiratory maneuver.

lung capacity (TLC) and then to exhale as forcefully as possible to residual volume (RV). [Horrific shrieks from the pulmonary function technologist usually help to provide incentive during the exhalation!] This creates a tracing like that shown in Figure 2–12. From the spirogram of the forced expiration maneuver one can see that the exhaled flow rate ($\Delta V/\Delta t$) is more rapid at the beginning of the exhalation than at the end, since the curve is steeper in the early part of the exhalation than the later.

It is useful to plot the instantaneous exhaled flow rate (liters/sec) as a function of exhaled volume. This is most easily done electronically, since the calculation of the slope by hand from the paper spirogram is tedious. Figure 2–13 is an example of such a plot of the instantaneous exhaled flow rate as a function of the volume of gas exhaled in a normal subject. Flows above the horizontal line are expiratory, while flows below the line are in an inspiratory direction. Lung volumes are greater toward the left side and lowest at the right side, since the volume being plotted on the x-axis is exhaled volume. The collection of small loops in the center was obtained during quiet tidal breathing. By inspection, the tidal volume in this subject averaged about 700 ml. During quiet breathing, the maximum flow encountered during inspiration or expiration was about 1 liter/sec, which is much lower than the maximum flow rates that the lung is capable of achieving. At the start of the maneuver, the subject inhaled

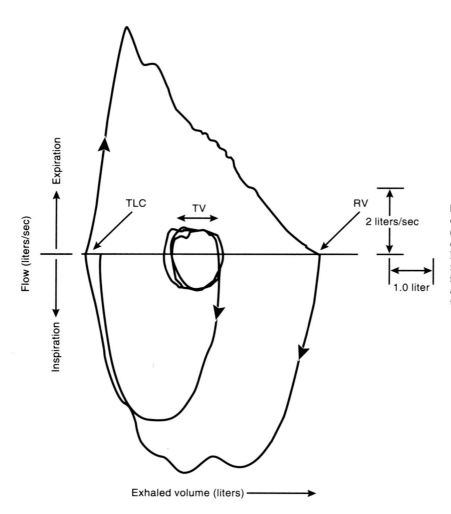

Figure 2–13. Air flow rate (on the ordinate) as a function of lung volume (on the abscissa) during a forced expiratory maneuver. Points above the horizontal axis represent expiratory flows; points below the line are inspiratory. Lung volumes are highest at the left and lowest at the right. See text for further explanation.

deeply and forcefully to TLC (large downward [inspiratory] flow beginning at FRC) and then immediately exhaled forcefully down to RV (large upward [expiratory] flow ending at RV). Several typical characteristics can be noted in this *flow–volume loop.*

First, note that the maximal inspiratory flow was about the same or greater than the maximal expiratory flow. The maximum inspiratory flow rate is influenced by several factors. On one hand, the maximum force that can be generated by the inspiratory muscles decreases as lung volume increases above RV. Hence, the inspiratory force decreases as inhalation proceeds. Second, the static recoil pressure of the lung increases as lung volume increases above RV. This opposes the inspiratory muscles and tends to reduce maximum inspiratory flow rate. On the other hand, airways resistance tends to decrease as lung volume increases because the caliber of the airways increases. Normally, the above factors

combine to cause maximal inspiratory flow to occur about halfway between TLC and RV. During forced expiration the flow rate rises rapidly at the start of the exhalation and reaches its peak early in the exhalation while lung volume is still high. Thereafter, the flow rate decreases progressively toward the end of the exhalation.

Figure 2–14 shows three flow-volume curves superimposed on the same graph. To generate these curves a subject performed three forced expirations, each with progressively greater effort. As the effort increases, note that the peak flow early in the expiration also increases. However, in the later part of the expiration all three curves converge, indicating that the flow rate in the later part of expiration is *effort independent.* In that range, the expiratory rate is *flow-limited* by the lung, and no amount of additional effort can increase the flow rate beyond this limit. Thus, over much of a forced expiration the maximal flow rate is determined by a property of

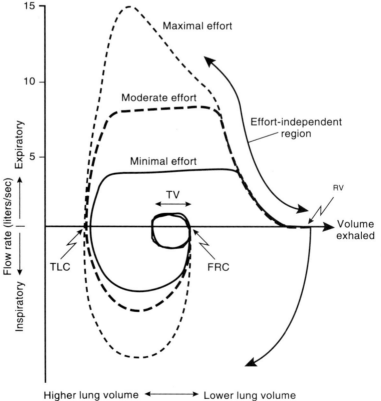

Figure 2–14. Three superimposed expiratory flow maneuvers, made with increasing effort. Note that peak inspiratory and expiratory flow rates are *effort dependent,* whereas expiratory flow rates later in expiration are *effort independent.*

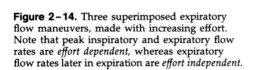

the lungs and not by the effort expended by the subject. This measurement is highly reproducible in a single subject and is relatively sensitive to changes in lung properties caused by diseases. Accordingly, the forced expiratory flow–volume loop has become a common clinical test of pulmonary function.

Lung Volume and Maximal Expiratory Flow Rate

During a forced exhalation, flow rate rises rapidly to a peak early in the maneuver but then decreases progressively as lung volume diminishes. In the effort-independent portion of the flow–volume relationship, the *maximal* expiratory flow rate in any given subject is heavily influenced by *lung volume*. This concept is shown graphically in Figure 2–15*A*. To generate this graph, a subject with an esophageal balloon catheter (to measure pleural pressure) was asked to exhale several times, with increasing effort. The first few exhalations were made with mild effort, while the subsequent exhalations were made with increasing effort, up to a maximal effort. During forceful exhalations, pleural pressure increased significantly (to 40–60 cm H_2O), while during less forceful exhalations the rise in pleural pressure was

less. During each exhalation, expiratory flow and exhaled volume were recorded *only when the lung volume passed through a predetermined level*. For example, consider the curve labeled 3 in Figure 2–15. This line represents the different flow rates measured during exhalations at different efforts, at the times that 70% of the vital capacity had been exhaled. Thus, the lung volumes corresponding to all of the points on curve 3 are identical. Similarly, the points on curve 4 represent the different expiratory flow rates that were obtained during exhalations of varying intensity, at the point where 90% of the vital capacity had been exhaled (i.e., lung volume = RV + 10% of VC). For curve 2, expiratory flow rate (at that lung volume) increases with increasing effort, until a maximal flow is reached. Further effort (higher pleural pressure) will not increase expiratory flow above the plateau value for that lung volume. Note that the maximal flow for curve 2 was greater than for curve 3, and the lung volume corresponding to 2 was greater than for 3. Thus, the maximum expiratory flow that can be achieved increases as the lung volume increases toward TLC. Another set of flows was collected at high lung volumes (90% of TLC) during various

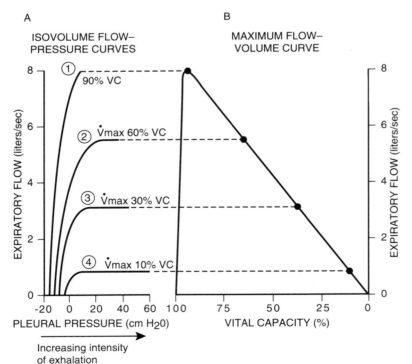

Figure 2–15. Greater levels of (effort-independent) expiratory flow rate can be achieved when lung volume is higher. Each curve represents the relationship between expiratory effort (pleural pressure) and expiratory flow rate *that would have been noted if lung volume could have remained constant*. At any given lung volume, expiratory flow rate increases with expiratory effort until an effort-independent expiratory flow rate is reached. Above this level, further increases in effort do not produce increases in flow rate. At total lung capacity in a normal subject, increases in effort always produce increases in flow rate. See text for further explanation. (Redrawn from Murray JF: The Normal Lung, 2nd ed. Philadelphia, WB Saunders, 1986.)

exhalations with varying effort (curve 1). Note that at this high lung inflation, expiratory flows continued to increase with increasing effort; that is, there was no clear limitation to flow other than effort. Since each of curves 1 through 4 correspond to specific lung volumes, these relationships are referred to as *isovolume pressure–flow curves.*

If the *maximal* values of expiratory flow (see Figure 2–15B) are plotted as a function of their respective lung volumes (volume below TLC), this yields a curve whose shape is identical to the descending portion of a single-breath forced-exhalation maneuver. Thus, the clinical measurement of a single forced exhalation provides (in the effort-independent region) a continuous plot of the maximal flow that can be achieved at lung volumes ranging from near TLC to RV.

Expiratory Flow Limitation Mechanism

As described previously, maximal expiratory flow rates are normally limited by factors other than effort after lung volume falls more than about 20% of the way from TLC toward RV. The reason for this is that airways are intrinsically floppy, distensible tubes that tend to become compressed when the pressure outside them exceeds the pressure inside. Stated more formally, airways become liable to collapse when their transmural pressure (defined as inside-minus-outside pressure difference) becomes negative. Expiratory flow-limitation occurs when highly localized events called *choke points* (not related to ordinary choking) occur at specific sites along the airways where negative transmural pressures cause a critical narrowing in the airway diameter. This is roughly analogous to the situation that occurs when attempting to drink water through a paper soda straw that has become saturated with water and is soggy and collapsible. If the subject draws too forcefully on the straw, the pressure inside becomes negative with respect to ambient pressure and the straw collapses. When this occurs, no amount of additional effort will cause the flow to increase. However, one can still draw water slowly through the straw without causing the flow limitation to occur.

Figure 2–16 shows the sequence of events that occur during expiratory flow limitation in a lung surrounded by the chest wall and the pleural space. Note that the airways are shown schematically as

tapered tubes, because the total airway cross-sectional area narrows enormously in traveling from the alveoli to the trachea. Figure 2–16A shows the lung held at TLC while no airflow is occurring. In this state, alveolar pressure is zero (relative to atmospheric) and pleural pressure is -30 cm H_2O, so the lung transmural pressure (transpulmonary pressure) equals $+30$ cm H_2O. Since there is no flow, the pressure inside the airways is also zero. Since the pressure immediately outside the intrathoracic airways is the same as pleural pressure, the transmural pressure (pressure inside–pressure outside) for the airways is also $+30$ cm H_2O. This positive transmural pressure tends to hold the airways open, in the same way that a positive transpulmonary pressure holds the alveoli open.

Next, consider what happens at the instant a forced exhalation begins (see Figure 2–16B). As the inspiratory muscles relax and expiratory muscles contract, the chest volume decreases and pleural pressure rises rapidly to $+60$ cm H_2O. At that instant, alveolar pressure rises to 90 cm H_2O, because alveolar pressure exceeds pleural pressure by the static lung recoil pressure corresponding to that lung volume. Driven by a pressure difference between alveolus and the mouth of 90 cm H_2O, expiratory flow begins in earnest. As expiratory flow begins, a gradient in pressure develops inside the airways between the alveoli and the mouth, as shown in Figure 2–16B. This reduces the transmural pressure for the airways, because it lowers the pressure in the lumen relative to the pressure outside the bronchi (pleural pressure). Two major factors contribute to the fall in intra-airway pressure between the alveoli and the mouth. First, there is a resistive pressure drop caused by the frictional pressure loss associated with the flow. This resistive loss becomes greater toward the trachea, because the number of parallel airways decreases more rapidly than the diameter of the individual airways increase (see Figure 2–3). The second factor lowering the pressure inside the airways is caused by the fact that the gas velocity increases toward the trachea, because the total cross-sectional area of the airways decreases. This acceleration of gas flow further decreases the pressure, due to the Bernoulli effect (see Figure 2–4). Both contributions tend to lower the airway transmural pressure, thereby decreasing the diameter of the airways. During the exhalation, lung volume decreases so the static re-

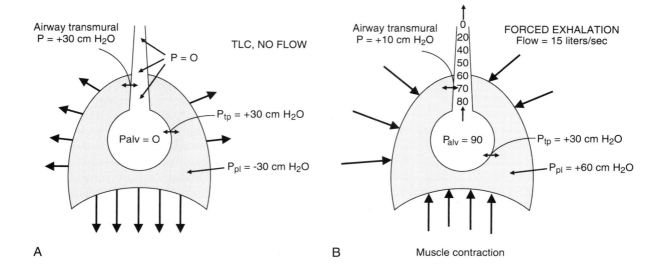

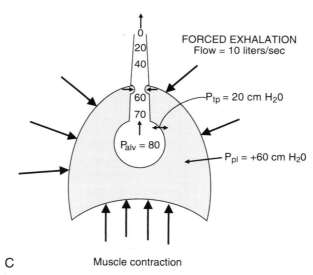

Figure 2–16. *A*, End inspiration, before the start of exhalation. *B*, At the start of a forced exhalation. *C*, Expiratory flow limitation later in a forced exhalation. Expiratory flow limitation occurs at locations where airway diameter is narrowed as a result of a negative transmural pressure. See text for further explanation.

coil pressure decreases. This lowers the difference between pleural pressure and alveolar pressure, thereby decreasing a major factor contributing to airway transmural pressure. In addition, the mechanical tethering (Figure 2–17) that helps to hold the airways open at high lung volumes becomes less as lung volume decreases. Moreover, the mainstem bronchi and the trachea are not surrounded by alveoli and therefore do not benefit from this support.

Figure 2–16C shows the balance of forces acting during expiratory flow-limitation. At this point, pleural pressure is still at 60 cm H_2O and lung volume has decreased by 20% from TLC. Lung static recoil pressure at this volume is +20 cm H_2O, so alveolar pressure is $20 + 60 = 80$ cm H_2O. Expiratory flow is 10 liters/sec, and the pressure inside the airways decreases from 80 cm H_2O (at the alveoli) to 0 cm H_2O (at the mouth). At the point where the

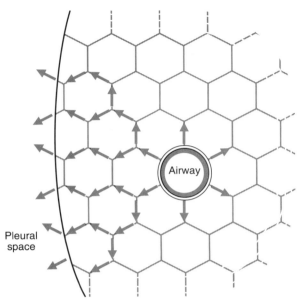

Figure 2–17. Airway tethering by the surrounding alveoli. At higher lung volumes there is more tension in the alveolar septal walls. This tension is transmitted to the airways passing through the lung parenchyma, tending to increase their diameter and prevent their collapse (*mechanical tethering*). Hence, higher expiratory flows can be achieved at high lung volumes.

pressure inside the airways has decreased to less than 60 cm H_2O (somewhere between the alveoli and the mouth), the pressure outside the airways becomes greater than the pressure inside. This negative airway transmural pressure causes the airway to narrow, as a choke point forms. For this reason, a greater expiratory effort (higher pleural pressure) cannot increase the flow further because the higher pleural pressure will tend to collapse the airway at the choke point just as much as it tends to increase the driving gradient for flow. This is why effort-independent expiratory flow limitation occurs in forced exhalation.

As expiration continues, lung static recoil pressure continues to decrease because lung volume decreases. The fall in static recoil pressure decreases the transmural pressure tending to hold the airways open, facilitating the development of a choke point. Airway resistance also increases at lower lung volumes, accentuating the resistive drop in pressure along the airways. Finally, mechanical tethering of the airways becomes less at lower lung volumes, thus promoting the collapse at a choke point. These

factors contribute to the lessened maximal expiratory flow that occurs later in a forced exhalation.

In summary, flow limitation occurs at specific sites of narrowing (choke points) along the airway, which are likely to form at locations where the airway transmural pressure becomes negative. The major factor contributing to a positive airway transmural pressure is a high lung static recoil pressure (high lung volume), because this contributes to a greater pressure within the airspaces relative to pleural pressure. Factors that tend to reduce airway transmural pressure during expiration (thus promoting flow-limitation) are (1) the resistive drop in pressure due to airflow from alveoli toward the mouth; (2) the Bernoulli reduction of intra-airway pressure caused by the acceleration of flow as the total airway cross-sectional area decreases toward the mouth; and (3) loss of mechanical tethering of central airways as they exit from the lung.

Tests of Expiratory Flow Limitation in Lung Diseases

The *vital capacity* (VC) measured as the change in volume from TLC to RV during a forced expiration is called the *forced vital capacity* (FVC). Line AB in the inset of Figure 2–12 connects the points on the FVC curve at 25% of VC and 75% of VC. This provides an "average slope" (liters/sec) in the middle of the forced expiration and is termed FEF_{25-75} (forced expiratory flow between 25% and 75% of FVC). This provides an index of the forced expiratory flow within the effort-independent (flow-limited) range. However, in practice there is considerable variability in this measurement among individuals. A more reproducible number is the volume of air (in liters) exhaled during the first second of the forced exhalation. This volume is termed the *forced expiratory volume in 1 second* (FEV_1). Typically, the FEV_1 is normalized by dividing it by the FVC and expressing the result as a percentage. Note that the FEV_1/FVC ratio is dimensionless, since it is the ratio of two dimensionally similar terms. In healthy persons between the ages of 25 and 50 the FEV_1/FVC is usually between 75% and 85%.

Acute and chronic lung diseases can change the expiratory flow–volume relationship by virtue of the changes they cause in (1) static lung recoil pressures; (2) airways resistance and the distribution of resistance along the airways; (3) loss of mechanical tethering of intraparenchymal airways; (4) changes in the stiffness or mechanical properties of the airways; and (5) regional differences in the severity of the above changes among lung regions.

Abnormally low values of FEV_1, FEF_{25-75}, and FEV_1/FVC are the hallmark of *obstructive lung diseases*. Diseases in this category include emphysema, asthma, chronic bronchitis, and cystic fibrosis. The common observation among these diverse diseases is that expiratory flow becomes limited at relatively low flow rates (hence the term *obstructive*), although the mechanism responsible varies among the diseases. In *asthma*, flow limitation occurs primarily as a result of decreased airway caliber caused by abnormally increased bronchial smooth muscle tone and swelling of the mucosal layer lining the airways. In *chronic bronchitis* and *cystic fibrosis*, the accumulation of excessive bronchial secretions hinders normal air flow. In *emphysema*, the decreased static lung recoil (increased lung compliance) resulting from the destruction of alveolar septal walls tends to promote the development of flow-limitation (choke points) at much lower flow rates than for normal persons. The loss in static recoil pressure also causes TLC to be increased, as is FRC. Accordingly, emphysematous patients often breathe at higher lung volumes than do normal subjects. Finally, the loss in elastic tethering of intraparenchymal airways further promotes the development of choke points during exhalation.

Figure 2–18 shows an expiratory flow–volume loop in a patient with emphysema. Compared with the normal subject, TLC and FRC are both increased. Note that during quiet tidal breathing, the emphysematous patient's expiratory curve intersects the maximal expiratory curve, indicating that resting exhalations in this patient are already flow limited! Note also that the shape of the expiratory curve is deeply convex owing to the severe flow limitation at lower lung volumes. By contrast, inspiratory flows are relatively normal, since the negative pleural pressure during inspiration tends to promote airway opening by increasing airway transmural pressures. Consequently, rapid inspiration is not a problem for these patients whereas exhalation is a slow and extended process.

Another class of lung diseases are termed *restrictive diseases*, because they restrict the extent of lung inflation. Decreased TLC is the hallmark of restrictive diseases, which generally arise from three different causes: (1) diseases causing increased static lung recoil such as *interstitial fibrosis*; (2) diseases limiting chest wall movement such as *kyphoscoliosis* or (more commonly) *obesity*; and (3) muscular weakness, such as in *myasthenia gravis*. The effect of restrictive disease on lung statics and dynamics varies with the cause and the extent of the disease.

Restrictive disease associated with an increased lung static recoil often occurs in pulmonary interstitial fibrosis. Compared with a normal subject, TLC and RV are both reduced, owing to the increased static lung recoil. Although maximal expiratory flows may appear to be increased in these patients (FEV_1/FVC ratio is elevated), the FEV_1 may be normal or even reduced, while FVC is significantly reduced. Thus, expiratory flows would not be elevated if plotted as a function of pleural pressure.

Features characteristic of restrictive lung disease are also associated with diseases involving muscle weakness. In these patients, TLC is low because there is insufficient strength to overcome the static recoil of the lungs and chest wall associated with a normal TLC. Likewise, RV may be high because there is insufficient strength to reach a normal RV. However, static lung recoil can be normal, so the expiratory flows are not elevated above normal.

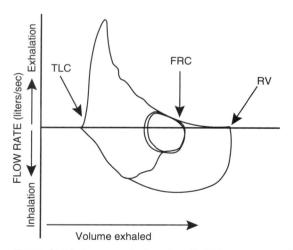

Figure 2–18. Severe expiratory flow limitation can occur in a patient with emphysema. This flow–volume loop shows that expiratory flow rate falls sharply after the start of expiration. The remainder of expiration is prolonged, owing to the slow rate of flow-limited exhalation. Note also the increased total lung capacity and increased functional residual capacity, caused by the increased lung compliance in this patient.

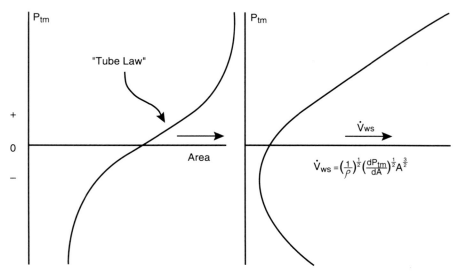

Figure 2–19. *Left,* Typical relationship between the cross-sectional area of an airway (A) and the transmural pressure across it (P_{tm}). When the transmural pressure across an airway is negative, the airway area decreases to a minimum level as the tube is squeezed shut. As P_{tm} increases, the airway assumes a more normal shape and its area increases. However, at high transmural pressures the airway elastic elements are stretched and further changes in area with increased transmural pressure are small. Flow limitation is more likely to occur in floppy airways because they tend to collapse more readily as their transmural pressure decreases. *Right,* The maximal flow that can develop in a floppy tube ($\dot{V}_{ws}$) depends on the stiffness of the tube: the more rigid the tube, the greater the maximal flow. (Redrawn from Mead J: Expiratory flow limitation: a physiologist's point of view. Fed Proc 39:2771, 1980.)

Restrictive diseases arising from decreases in chest wall compliance can reduce FRC because lung static recoil is unchanged while static chest wall recoil is increased. The increased chest wall recoil can also lead to a decrease in TLC because the maximal decrease in pleural pressure that can be developed by the respiratory muscles will not increase lung volume to a normal TLC.

Physics of Expiratory Flow Limitation

Effort-independent expiratory flow limitation occurs at points along the airways where the local transmural pressure is negative enough to cause the airway to narrow, causing the appearance of a choke point that limits the flow rate. If the airways were stiff, rigid tubes, then choke points would not occur because the caliber of the airways would remain fixed over a wide range of transmural pressures. Real airways are not rigid but can vary in their degree of stiffness at different locations (i.e., trachea vs. small bronchi), depending on how much carti-

lage is present, what surrounds the airway at that point, and other factors. Hence, some points along the airway are more likely to form choke points than others.

In floppy tubes such as airways, the maximum flow that can occur at any point is related to the product of the velocity of propagation of a pressure wave along the tube (the *tube wave speed*), and the cross-sectional area of the tube at that point. This theoretical maximum flow is called the *tube wave speed flow* ($\dot{V}ws$):

$$\dot{V}ws = \left[\frac{1}{\rho} \cdot \frac{dP_{tm}}{dA} \right]^{\frac{1}{2}} \cdot A^{\frac{3}{2}}$$

where ρ is the gas density, A is the tube cross-sectional area at that point, and dP_{tm}/dA is related to the elasticity of the tube. Figure 2–19 shows a typical relationship between the area of an airway (A) and the transmural pressure across it (P_{tm}). When the transmural pressure across an airway is negative, the airway area decreases to a minimum level. As P_{tm} increases, the airway assumes a more normal shape and its area increases. However, at high transmural pressures, the airway elastic elements are stretched and further changes in area with increased transmural pressure are small. The dP_{tm}/dA term in the equation is the slope of this relationship at any given point. This curve is sometimes called the *tube law,* since it describes how the area of a specific tube will vary with transmural pressure. The above formula states that if the stiffness of an airway is known (i.e., the tube law) and if the density of the gas is known, then the maximum

theoretical flow that can occur in that airway is known. Factors that tend to increase the area of an airway (i.e., parenchymal tethering at high lung volumes) or that make an airway wall less floppy (i.e., more cartilage) tend to increase the maximum theoretical flow that the airway can support ($\dot{V}ws$). As the actual flow in an airway increases, it reaches a maximum when it equals the wave speed flow. Above that maximum flow a choke point forms, and flow is limited to the maximum value. This approach to understanding the physical mechanisms underlying expiratory flow limitation is termed *wave speed theory.*

Chapter 3

Ventilation

Ventilation is the process by which fresh gas is brought into the respiratory system to replace a portion of the gas it contains. In mammals this is accomplished by a periodic pattern of breathing called *tidal ventilation.* In the process, carbon dioxide is eliminated from the body in exhaled gas and oxygen is brought into the lungs to replace the oxygen taken up from the airspaces into the blood. Ventilation is normally maintained by the action of the respiratory muscles under the control of the respiratory control centers in the medulla oblongata region of the brain.

The Respiratory Muscles

Ventilation is normally achieved by coordinated contraction of specific muscle groups, whose action serves to increase and decrease the volume of the thoracic cavity. Inspiration is normally an active process that requires contraction of the diaphragm and other muscle groups that are referred to as the *inspiratory muscles.* The muscles of respiration are skeletal muscles that exhibit structural, electrical, and functional characteristics that are identical with other skeletal muscles. In this regard, the force of contraction developed by the respiratory muscles increases when they are stretched to a greater initial length and decreases when their initial length is relatively shorter. Since a change in lung volume (e.g., functional residual capacity [FRC]) affects the lengths of the respiratory muscle groups, it also affects the forces that those muscles can develop.

The primary muscle of inspiration is the *diaphragm,* which is composed of three primary muscle fiber types (slow oxidative, fast glycolytic, and fast oxidative glycolytic), and is innervated bilaterally by the phrenic nerve. The diaphragm forms a highly curved basal floor of the thoracic cavity. It inserts into the lower ribs and the sternum anteriorly and the spine posteriorly. By the law of LaPlace, increased tension in the curved diaphragm causes a pressure difference between the thorax and abdomen, forcing the abdominal contents downward as the thoracic volume increases. If not for this curvature, contraction of the diaphragm would be less effective at increasing thoracic volume.

The *external intercostal muscles* are located between the ribs and tend to lift the rib cage superiorly and laterally during inspiration. This motion increases the angle between the ribs and the spine, thereby increasing thoracic volume. Figure 3–1 shows this change, which increases both the anteroposterior and the lateral dimensions of the chest wall during inspiration. The *parasternal intercostal muscles* are particularly effective in this regard, especially under conditions in which breathing is labored. Like the diaphragm, the intercostal muscles are composed of three primary muscle fiber types.

The *scalenus muscles* insert into the first rib and help to elevate the ribs during inspiration. These muscles are often active even during quiet breathing. Other *accessory muscles* of inspiration include the *sternocleidomastoid muscle*, which inserts into the sternum and helps to elevate the rib cage during inspiration. The *trapezius muscles*, the *major and minor pectoralis muscles*, the *serrati muscles*, and others also contribute to ventilation when the work

of breathing is increased. In addition, the *abdominal muscles* help to facilitate inspiration by compressing the abdominal contents during posture movements, which helps to maintain the diaphragm at a more optimum length.

At rest, exhalation is normally passive and is accomplished by relaxing the inspiratory muscles. This allows the elastic (potential) energy stored in the lung and chest wall to return the lung to its end-expiratory volume. When ventilation is increased (as in exercise) or the work of breathing is increased (as may occur in lung diseases), specific muscle groups contribute actively to expiration. During active expiration, the muscles of the abdominal wall compress the abdominal contents inward, forcing the relaxing diaphragm upward into the chest. These muscles include the *rectus abdominus, transverse abdominus,* and the *internal and external oblique muscles.* The *internal intercostal muscles* also contribute to exhalation by pulling the rib cage downward and decreasing the anteroposterior and lateral dimensions of the rib cage.

Respiratory Muscles in Diseases

Different diseases can affect ventilation by affecting the mechanical properties of the lungs or chest wall or by influencing the ability of the respiratory muscles to contract normally. In diseases in which the workload of the respiratory muscles is increased abruptly (e.g., during acute *asthma*), little opportunity is available for adaptation of the muscles. In this setting, *acute ventilatory failure* may result abruptly as the respiratory muscles fatigue under the added workload. Mechanical ventilation is used clinically to support patients in danger of developing acute ventilatory failure. During mechanical ventilation, the ventilator takes over the work of the respiratory muscles, thus maintaining normal ventilation while allowing the muscles to rest and permitting the acute condition responsible for the increased work of breathing to resolve.

In *chronic obstructive lung disease* the work of breathing is increased by the airflow obstruction. Moreover, the increase in total lung capacity in emphysema is associated with a downward movement of the diaphragm. This shortens the muscle fibers of the diaphragm and reduces its radius of curvature. Both of these factors contribute to a reduced ability of the diaphragm to function normally and may

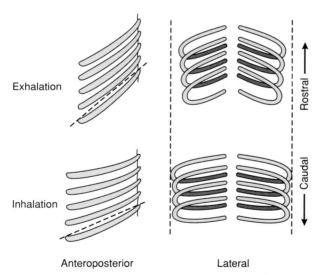

Figure 3–1. Chest wall dimensions. Contraction of the diaphragm causes the basal floor of the thoracic cavity to move downward, displacing the abdominal contents downward and increasing the rostral-caudal dimensions of the thoracic cavity. Contractions of the external intercostal muscles, the scalenus muscles, and the sternocleidomastoid muscles lift the rib cage superiorly and laterally, increasing the anteroposterior and the lateral dimensions of the chest wall.

Exhalation

Inhalation

Anteroposterior

Lateral

Rostral

Caudal

contribute to respiratory muscle fatigue. In diseases in which lung stiffness is increased acutely such as in severe *pulmonary edema,* the increased load on the respiratory muscles may likewise contribute to respiratory muscle fatigue. In patients with the neuromuscular disease *poliomyelitis* the function of the major muscles of inspiration may be impaired while the function of certain accessory muscle groups (such as the sternocleidomastoids) may remain normal. These patients can frequently maintain ventilation for extended periods of time using the accessory muscles alone, which become enlarged (hypertrophied) over time under the workload. In neuromuscular diseases such as *Guillain-Barré* syndrome or *myasthenia gravis,* weakness of the respiratory muscles can lead to acute respiratory failure even though the mechanical properties of the lung and chest wall may remain normal (i.e., the work of breathing is normal).

COMPOSITION OF AMBIENT, INSPIRED, AND EXPIRED GASES

In studying the function of the lung as a gas exchange organ, it is useful to begin by considering the properties of gases involved in ventilation. Atmospheric air is a mixture of oxygen, nitrogen, argon, and trace quantities of other gases, including carbon dioxide. Table 3–1 shows the composition of ambient air. Note that all of the *dry gas fractions* present in a mixture must sum to a total of 1.0. The composition of a gas mixture can be described in terms of either the gas fractions or the corresponding *partial pressures*. The partial pressure of a single gas within a mixture is that portion of the total pressure contributed by that gas. Hence, the partial pressure of a gas is calculated as the product of the *dry gas fraction* and the total ambient *(barometric)* pressure (P_{baro}):

$$P_{gas} = P_{baro} \cdot F_{gas}$$

Thus, if the barometric pressure is 760 torr at sea level, then the ambient oxygen partial pressure would be

$$760 \cdot 0.2093 = 159 \text{ torr.}$$

Table 3-1 also shows the partial pressures (or *tensions*) of the various gases in ambient air, assuming a barometric pressure of 760 torr. Since each of the gases present contributes part of the total barometric pressure, the sum of all the gas partial pressures must equal the total barometric pressure. At high altitude the gas fractions of ambient air are the same as at sea level, but the barometric pressure is lower. Hence, the partial pressures of all ambient gases decrease at high altitude even though their gas fractions remain the same.

TABLE 3–1
Gas Partial Pressures in Ambient Air, Inspired Air, and Alveolar Gas

Gas	Dry Ambient Air		Inspired Air*	Alveolar Gas*
	Fraction	Gas Tension	Gas Tension	Gas Tension
Nitrogen	0.7809	593.5	556.8	566
Oxygen	0.2093	159.1	149.2	100
Carbon dioxide	0.0003	0.23	0.21	40
Argon and other inert gases	0.0095	7.2	6.8	6.9
Water	0	0	47	47
Total	1.00	760	760	760

*Assumes body temperature of 37°C and a barometric pressure of 760 torr. All gas partial pressures are expressed in torr.

E X A M P L E. Calculate the ambient oxygen tension at the summit of Mt. Whitney if the barometric pressure is 450 torr.

$$P_{O_2} = P_{baro} \cdot F_{O_2}$$

$$P_{O_2} = 450 \cdot 0.2093 = 94.2 \text{ torr} \quad \blacksquare$$

As gas is inhaled it comes into contact with the moist, warm epithelial surface lining the nasopharynx and upper airways, where it becomes humidified and warmed to body temperature. En route to the alveoli the inspired gas becomes *saturated* with water vapor, meaning that it takes up as much water as it can hold at that temperature. Gas saturated with water has a *water vapor partial pressure* that depends on the temperature. At body temperature (37°C), saturated gas has a constant water vapor partial pressure of 47 torr. By providing 47 torr toward the total barometric pressure, the addition of water effectively reduces the partial pressures of the other gases present, even before they reach the alveoli. Table 3–1 also shows the composition of *inspired air*, defined as ambient air that has been inhaled *but has not yet reached the lung alveoli.* Note that the process of saturating dry ambient air during inspiration produces a 10 torr decrease in the P_{O_2} of gas before it even reaches the alveoli. In practice, ambient air normally does contain some moisture. However, this is usually small (e.g., the ambient water vapor partial pressure at 20°C is 17.5 torr if the air is saturated and less if the relative humidity is less than 100%). The important concept is that to correctly calculate a gas partial pressure in a humidified mixture, the water vapor partial pressure should first be subtracted from the total barometric pressure.

E X A M P L E. Calculate the ambient and inspired nitrogen partial pressure for a subject riding in a commercial jet airplane where the cabin is pressurized to 550 torr. (Ambient air in a commercial airliner can be assumed to be very dry.)

Ambient air contains 78.1% nitrogen, so

$$\text{ambient } P_{N_2} = 550 \cdot 0.781 = 429.6 \text{ torr.}$$

Inspired gas is humidified to a partial pressure of 47 torr, so

$$P_{IN_2} = (550 - 47) \cdot 0.781 = 392.8 \text{ torr.} \quad \blacksquare$$

LUNG VENTILATION

Figure 3–2*A* shows a schematic diagram of the airway tree as it branches sequentially from the trachea toward the alveolar sacs. In this model, an airway generation is defined in terms of the number of branch points encountered, with the trachea labeled as generation 0, the mainstem bronchi as generation 1, and so on. Anatomical studies have identified about 23 to 27 generations of branching in the lung. Airways in humans generally branch *dichotomously* into two equally sized daughter branches. Functionally, airways can be classified into two major zones. The first is referred to as the *conducting zone,* because it is composed entirely of airways that serve only to conduct gas between the lung periphery and the mouth. The second is termed the *respiratory zone* since airways in this zone directly give rise to alveoli that participate in gas exchange. The conducting zone comprises about the first 15 to 17 generations of airways, whereas the respiratory zone comprises the remaining generations down to the alveoli. (See also Chapter 12.)

Figure 3–2*B* shows the relative gas volumes of the conducting and respiratory zones of the lung. At FRC, an adult human lung contains about 3 liters of gas. Most of the gas volume is contained in alveoli, whereas only 100 to 200 ml is contained in the conducting airways. (An approximate rule of thumb is that the volume of the conducting airways is approximately equal to the body weight expressed in pounds.) (Figure 3–3.) During inspiration, lung volume rises by the *tidal volume* (V_T). Note that since the volume of the conducting airways increases relatively little during inspiration of a 500-ml tidal volume, the increase in *alveolar volume* during the breath will be nearly 500 ml. However, note that the first gas to enter the alveoli at the beginning of an inspiration will have been the gas that remained in the airways at the end of the previous exhalation. This is not fresh gas; it is gas that exited from alveoli during the previous breath.

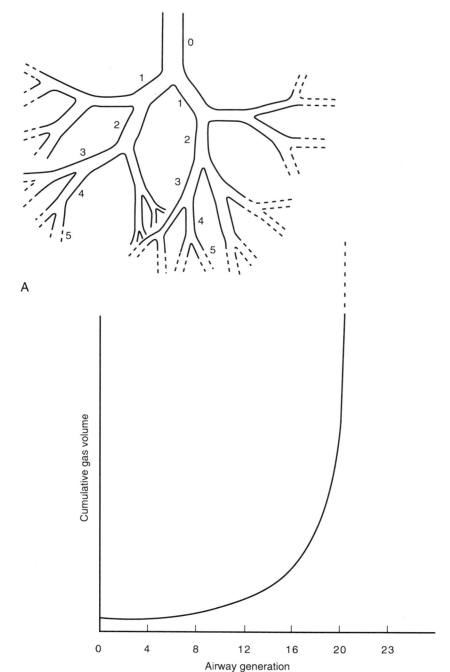

Figure 3-2. *A*. Branching pattern of the airways from the trachea to the alveoli. Airway generations are defined according to the number of branching points encountered, with the trachea defined as generation 0. Approximately 23 to 27 generations of branching are encountered in the lung. The conducting zone of the lung encompasses those airway generations that only participate in gas transport. The respiratory zone of the lung begins at about generation 16 and contains airways that directly give rise to alveoli. (Redrawn from Weibel, 1960). *B*. Gas volumes contained in airways of different generations. The total gas volume in the conducting airways of an adult human averages 100 to 200 ml, while the average gas volume in the respiratory zone of the lungs averages 3000 to 4000 ml at functional residual capacity.

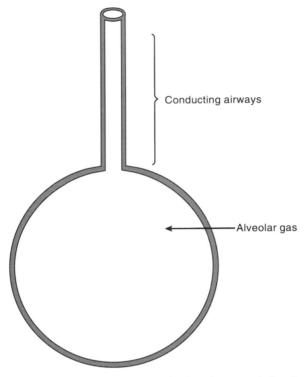

Conducting airways

Alveolar gas

Figure 3–3. Gas volumes in conducting airways and alveoli. Most of the gas contained in the lung at functional residual capacity (typically 3 liters) is in alveoli, whereas only 100 to 200 ml resides in the conducting airways. During a 500-ml inspiration, alveolar volume increases by nearly 500 ml, since the volume of the conducting airways increases little. However, not all of this is fresh alveolar ventilation since the first gas to enter the alveoli during a breath is the gas left in the conducting airways at the end of the previous exhalation.

Therefore, if the volume within the conducting airways is 150 ml and the tidal volume is 500 ml, only 350 ml of fresh gas will enter the alveoli with each inhalation. If the total alveolar gas volume at FRC is 3 liters, this 350 ml will change the alveolar gas composition by less than 12%. Because the amount of fresh gas entering the alveoli during quiet breathing is relatively small compared with the alveolar volume, the composition of alveolar gas is not dramatically altered over the course of a breath.

The product of the VT and the number of breaths per minute *(respiratory frequency)* is termed *minute volume (minute ventilation* or *total ventilation* [$\dot{V}E$]). Thus, with a normal respiratory frequency of 15 breaths per minute and a tidal volume of 500 ml, the minute ventilation would be 7500 ml/min. *Alveolar ventilation* ($\dot{V}A$) is defined as that portion of the minute ventilation that goes to ventilating alveoli that participate in gas exchange. The portion of the minute ventilation that does not contribute to alveolar ventilation is termed *anatomical dead space ventilation.*

E X A M P L E. If the volume of the conducting airways in a subject is 200 ml, the VT is 500 ml, and the respiratory frequency is 15 breaths per minute, calculate the alveolar ventilation and the anatomical dead space ventilation.

Alveolar ventilation will be the product of frequency and (VT minus dead space volume), or

$$15(500 - 200) = 4500 \ \text{ml/min.}$$

Anatomical dead space ventilation will be the product of dead space volume and frequency, or

$$200(15) = 3000 \ \text{ml/min.} \quad \blacksquare$$

ALVEOLAR VENTILATION AND CARBON DIOXIDE ELIMINATION

Strictly speaking, pulmonary ventilation is not continuous since it is accomplished by tidal breathing. Blood flow in the capillaries is not continuous either, since it speeds up during cardiac systole and may cease briefly during diastole. However, for the purposes of analysis it is useful to think of the lung *as if* it received a continuous flow of ventilation ($\dot{V}E$, liters/min) and a continuous blood flow (Q, liters/min), as shown in Figure 3–4. In this model of the lung, alveolar ventilation ($\dot{V}A$) is represented as a continuous gas flow through *alveoli that exchange gas with pulmonary capillary blood.* Anatomical dead space ventilation ($\dot{V}D$) contributes to the minute ventilation but does not contribute to alveolar ventilation. In effect, anatomical dead space ventilation bypasses the alveolar compartment.

Blood returning to the lungs from the rest of the body carries carbon dioxide produced by interme-

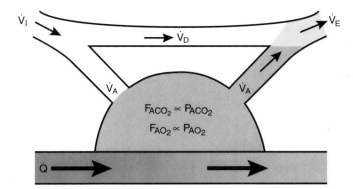

Figure 3–4. Continuous flow model of the lung. It is useful to think of the lung as if it received a continuous minute ventilation ($\dot{V}_E$) equal to the product of tidal volume and respiratory frequency. Alveolar ventilation ($\dot{V}_A$) is that part of $\dot{V}_E$ that travels to alveoli that participate in gas exchange. Anatomical dead space ventilation ($\dot{V}_D$) is the part of $\dot{V}_E$ that goes to ventilate conducting airways, and so effectively bypasses the alveoli.

diary metabolism in the cells. Some of this carbon dioxide leaves the blood as it passes through alveolar capillaries, and enters alveolar gas. The remainder of the carbon dioxide never leaves the blood and exits from the lung in pulmonary venous blood. The carbon dioxide that enters alveolar gas is eventually carried out of the lungs by alveolar ventilation. Under normal (steady state) conditions the volume of carbon dioxide produced by the cells of the body each minute ($\dot{V}_{CO_2}$, in ml/min) is equal to the volume of carbon dioxide eliminated from the lungs by alveolar ventilation ($\dot{V}_{CO_2}$, in ml/min). Note that if inspired gas contains no carbon dioxide, then the exhaled flow of carbon dioxide ($\dot{V}_{CO_2}$) must equal the product of alveolar ventilation ($\dot{V}_A$) and the fraction of $\dot{V}_A$ that is carbon dioxide:

$$\dot{V}_{CO_2} = \dot{V}_A \cdot F_{ACO_2}$$

where F_{ACO_2} is the dry gas fraction of carbon dioxide in alveolar gas. This is defined as the *alveolar carbon dioxide equation*. Stated alternatively, the carbon dioxide concentration in alveolar gas represents a balance between the rate of carbon dioxide production by the body ($\dot{V}_{CO_2}$) and the rate at which alveolar ventilation ($\dot{V}_A$) washes carbon dioxide out. This equation can be solved for the alveolar P_{CO_2}

(P_{ACO_2}), since

$$P_{ACO_2} = F_{ACO_2} \cdot (P_{baro} - P_{H_2O})$$

Thus,

$$P_{ACO_2} = \frac{\dot{V}_{CO_2}(P_{baro} - P_{H_2O})}{\dot{V}_A}.$$

The significance of this relationship is that alveolar P_{CO_2} is set by the ratio of carbon dioxide production to the alveolar ventilation. This relationship is shown graphically in Figure 3–5. For a given metabolic production of carbon dioxide, changes in alveolar ventilation produce reciprocal changes in alveolar P_{CO_2}. Hence, doubling alveolar ventilation will halve the alveolar P_{CO_2}, whereas doubling the metabolic production of carbon dioxide at constant alveolar ventilation will double alveolar P_{CO_2}. Since blood leaving the alveoli will normally have the same P_{CO_2} as alveolar gas, the P_{CO_2} in (what will become) systemic arterial blood is therefore determined by the level of alveolar ventilation, relative to the level of metabolic activity. Normally, the respiratory control centers in the brain stem regulate minute ventilation in accord with the level of $\dot{V}_{CO_2}$

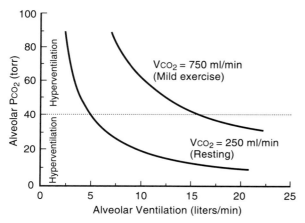

Figure 3 – 5. Alveolar P_{CO_2} as a function of alveolar ventilation in the lung. Each line corresponds to a given metabolic rate associated with a constant production of carbon dioxide ($\dot{V}_{CO_2}$ isometabolic line). Normally, alveolar ventilation is controlled to maintain an alveolar P_{CO_2} of about 40 torr. During *hypoventilation* the alveolar ventilation is low relative to $\dot{V}_{CO_2}$, and alveolar P_{CO_2} rises. During *hyperventilation* the alveolar ventilation is excessive relative to $\dot{V}_{CO_2}$ so the alveolar P_{CO_2} falls.

to control alveolar P_{CO_2} at about 40 torr. Specialized chemoreceptors monitor the P_{CO_2} in arterial blood and the brain stem and provide feedback information to the respiratory control centers regarding the P_{CO_2} in blood. Increases or decreases in systemic arterial P_{CO_2} elicit increases or decreases in minute ventilation in an attempt to maintain a normal alveolar P_{CO_2} (see Chapter 8). Increased P_{CO_2} in arterial blood can cause *respiratory acidosis,* whereas an abnormally low P_{CO_2} can produce *respiratory alkalosis.* Because abnormal blood pH values produced during these acid – base disorders can disrupt enzymatic and cellular function, the body attempts to control pH by regulating the alveolar P_{CO_2}. Thus, the cause of *hypercapnia* (elevated arterial P_{CO_2}) is inadequate alveolar ventilation relative to $\dot{V}_{CO_2}$ *(hypoventilation).* Conversely, *hyperventilation* exists when the alveolar ventilation is excessive with respect to metabolic production of carbon dioxide, leading to a low arterial P_{CO_2} *(hypocapnia).*

ANATOMICAL DEAD SPACE VENTILATION

The term *dead space* arises from the fact that this ventilation is wasted because it does not participate

in gas exchange. The *dead space to tidal volume ratio* (V_D/V_T) is defined as the volume of the anatomical dead space divided by the tidal volume. This ratio is a measure of how much of the minute ventilation is wasted in ventilating the conducting airways. Thus, *dead space ventilation* is the product of the minute ventilation ($\dot{V}_E$) and the dead space to tidal volume ratio (V_D/V_T):

$$\dot{V}_D = \frac{V_D}{V_T} \cdot \dot{V}_E.$$

Since the *volume* of the conducting airways changes relatively little over the course of a breath, the dead space ventilation varies inversely with the tidal volume. Thus, for the same minute ventilation the alveolar ventilation will be larger relative to dead space ventilation if the tidal volume is large and respiratory frequency is small, as opposed to using a small tidal volume and high frequency. Note also that doubling the minute ventilation normally will not double alveolar ventilation, since some portion of the minute ventilation is wasted as dead space ventilation. Normally, dead space ventilation represents 20 to 30% of the minute ventilation.

PHYSIOLOGICAL DEAD SPACE VENTILATION

As discussed above, anatomical dead space ventilation corresponds to the effective ventilation of lung regions that do not participate in gas exchange. In real lungs, and especially in diseased lungs, some alveoli may be excessively ventilated relative to others. When this happens the excessive ventilation is effectively wasted, even though it does travel to alveoli that participate in gas exchange. The *physiological dead space* ventilation refers to the total amount of wasted ventilation, including that due to the anatomical dead space as well as any wasted in excessively ventilated alveoli. Hence, the physiological dead space ventilation is at least as large as the anatomical dead space ventilation but may greatly exceed this value if many alveoli are excessively ventilated relative to others. In healthy individuals, the physiological dead space normally represents 25% to 35% of the minute ventilation.

A common technique to measure physiological dead space makes use of the fact that wasted ventilation does not effectively participate in gas ex-

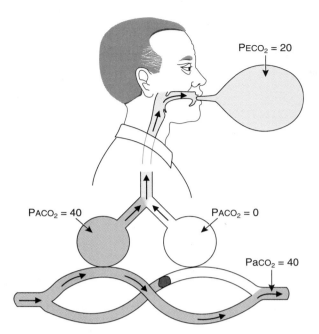

Figure 3-6. Physiological dead space can be determined by measuring the P_{CO_2} in alveolar gas and in mixed expired gas. The dilution of carbon dioxide in mixed expired gas, relative to alveolar gas, provides a functional measure of the amount of wasted ventilation relative to the minute ventilation. Dead space 50% (0.5) in this example.

(Labels in figure: $P_{ECO_2} = 20$; $P_{ACO_2} = 40$; $P_{ACO_2} = 0$; $P_{aCO_2} = 40$*)*

change. Figure 3-6 shows a lung composed of conducting airways and two different subpopulations of alveoli. One alveolar population receives ventilation and blood flow, while the second group of alveoli receives ventilation but no blood flow. The carbon dioxide concentration in the first group is normal and approximately the same as the systemic arterial P_{CO_2}. By contrast, the P_{CO_2} in the *unperfused* (i.e., no blood flow) group of alveoli is zero, since no carbon dioxide enters these units from the blood. If the exhaled gas from this lung is collected in a bag

over a few minutes, the P_{CO_2} in the mixture will be less than the P_{CO_2} in the normal alveoli, since the carbon dioxide leaving these alveoli has become diluted by the gas leaving the conducting airways and the unperfused alveoli. If the P_{CO_2} in the perfused alveoli (P_{ACO_2}) is known and if the *mixed expired* P_{CO_2} (P_{ECO_2}) is measured, the physiological dead space can be calculated from the relationship

$$\frac{\dot{V}_D}{\dot{V}_T} = 1 - \frac{P_{ECO_2}}{P_{ACO_2}}.$$

This relationship was originally described by the physiologist Christian Bohr (1856–1923), and it is sometimes referred to as the *Bohr dead space*. It was later recognized that the arterial P_{CO_2} (P_{aCO_2}) could be substituted for the alveolar P_{ACO_2}, since these values are usually nearly equal:

$$\frac{\dot{V}_D}{\dot{V}_T} = 1 - \frac{P_{ECO_2}}{P_{aCO_2}}$$

Note the standard convention of using an (upper case) ''A'' to refer to alveolar gas and a (lower case) ''a'' to refer to arterial blood.

E X A M P L E. The expired gas from a subject is collected in a large floppy bag over a 3-minute period. The P_{ECO_2} in this mixture is found to be 30 torr. At the same time, an arterial blood sample reveals an arterial P_{CO_2} of 40 torr. What is the physiological dead space in this subject?

Substituting the arterial P_{CO_2} for the alveolar P_{CO_2},

$$\frac{\dot{V}_D}{\dot{V}_T} = 1.0 - \frac{30}{40} = 0.25$$

Thus, 25% of the minute ventilation in this subject did not participate in gas exchange. ■

Chapter 4

The Pulmonary Circulation

The *systemic circulation* is that part of the vascular system supplied by the left ventricle, which pumps blood through the aortic valve into the aorta (Figure 4–1). Large arteries branch off the aorta, supplying blood to different regions of the body. These large arteries branch progressively into smaller and smaller arteries, which eventually give rise to arterioles. The arterioles are the major site of blood flow resistance and therefore regulate the distribution of capillary blood flow among and within the organ systems of the body. As blood travels through the capillaries, it exchanges respiratory gases, nutrients, water, and metabolic products with the organ. After leaving the capillaries, blood returns to the heart through the venous system, which empties into the right atrium from the vena cava.

The *pulmonary circulation* refers to the vascular system that conducts blood from the right side of the heart through the lungs (Figure 4–1). Blood travels from the right atrium of the heart into the right ventricle by way of the tricuspid valve. The right ventricle ejects blood through the pulmonic valve into the pulmonary artery, which branches into lobar arteries supplying the major lobes of the lung. The lobar arteries enter the lung at the hilum and branch progressively into sublobar, segmental, subsegmental, and lobular arteries. The pulmonary alveolar septal capillaries travel within the alveolar walls, providing a large surface area available for equilibration between blood and alveolar gas. After passing through the capillaries, blood travels through the pulmonary venous system. Pulmonary veins converge toward the hilum of the lung, where they exit as lobar veins. The lobar veins all converge near the entrance to the left atrium.

Unlike the systemic circulation, arterial blood in the pulmonary circulation is relatively deoxygenated, while blood in the pulmonary veins is well

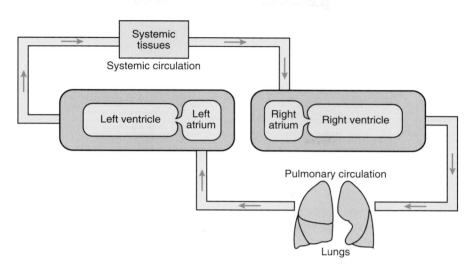

Figure 4-1. Pulmonary and systemic circulations. Blood flow exiting from the left ventricle through the aortic valve enters the systemic circulation, which returns the blood to the right atrium. Blood leaving the right ventricle through the pulmonic valve enters the pulmonary circulation, which returns blood to the left atrium.

oxygenated. Note that the entire cardiac output passes through both the systemic and pulmonary circulations each minute, since the two vascular systems operate in parallel. The blood volumes pumped through the pulmonary and systemic circulations over time must be equal; otherwise blood would progressively accumulate in either the pulmonary or systemic circulation. However, small differences between left- and right-sided heart outputs can occur briefly, over the course of one or two heart beats.

PRESSURES, VOLUMES, AND FLOWS IN THE PULMONARY CIRCULATION

The average hydrostatic pressure in the pulmonary artery is normally about 18 torr, compared with about 100 torr in systemic arteries. This difference is due to the low vascular resistance in the pulmonary bed relative to the systemic bed. The *vascular resistance* can be calculated from the difference between upstream and downstream pressures divided by the blood flow (cardiac output, $\dot{Q}t$):

$$PVR = \frac{(P1 - P2)}{\dot{Q}t}$$

The upstream pressure (P1) is the pulmonary arterial pressure, the downstream pressure (P2) is left

atrial pressure, and PVR is the pulmonary vascular resistance.

E X A M P L E. If cardiac output is 5 liters/min, calculate the pulmonary and systemic vascular resistances when mean pulmonary arterial pressure is 18 torr, mean systemic arterial pressure is 100 torr, right atrial pressure is 2 torr, and left atrial pressure is 5 torr.

For the lung, upstream pressure is 18, while downstream pressure is 5. Thus, PVR is

$$(18 - 5)/5 = 2.6 \text{ torr}/(\text{liter}/\text{min}).$$

For the systemic circulation, upstream pressure is 100 while downstream pressure is 2, so systemic vascular resistance is

$$(100 - 2)/5 = 19.6 \text{ torr}/(\text{liter}/\text{min}). \qquad \blacksquare$$

The pressure in the pulmonary circulation varies between a systolic value (typically 30 to 35 torr) and a diastolic value (typically 7 to 12 torr); its mean value is typically about 18 torr. Because its *pulse pressure* (systolic-diastolic pressure difference) is large relative to its mean pressure, the pulmonary circulation is highly pulsatile, compared with the systemic circulation. The volume of blood in the pulmonary circulation is small, compared with the systemic circulation. An adult human will typically have less than 500 ml of blood in the pulmonary vascular bed, of which about 75 ml is within the capillaries. By contrast, the systemic circulation in the same subject would normally contain more than 4 liters of blood.

Compared with the systemic circulation, the pulmonary circulation is a low pressure, low resistance vascular bed. The right ventricle is not normally capable of developing the high systolic pressures seen in the left ventricle, because its muscle mass is smaller. In addition, the geometry of the right ventricle (somewhat like a flat bellows attached to the side of the massive left ventricle) is less well suited to developing high pressures. However, the low pressure in the pulmonary circulation is still adequate to ensure that blood flow is distributed to all regions of the lung. The hydrostatic pressures in the pulmonary circulation are less than in the systemic circulation, and the pulmonary arteries contain much less smooth muscle than systemic arteries of equivalent size. Pulmonary arteries course through the lung tissue (*parenchyma*) adjacent to the bronchi, whereas the pulmonary veins returning to the lung hilum travel by a different route. If it were not for this anatomical distinction, it would be difficult to distinguish pulmonary arteries from veins, because both contain relatively little smooth muscle.

Pulmonary alveolar septal capillaries have a large surface area relative to their blood volume, which facilitates their function of gas exchange (Figure 4–2). Since they surround the alveoli and contain little in the way of structural reinforcement, the caliber of the capillaries is highly sensitive to the shape and size of the alveoli. Hence, the diameter of pulmonary capillaries depends heavily on their *transmural pressure* (inside-outside pressure difference). For example, if the volume of an alveolus is increased, the stretch and distortion of the alveolar wall narrows the capillaries and decreases their blood volume. This distortion causes an increase in its resistance to blood flow relative to that in normally inflated alveoli. Likewise, if capillary hydrostatic pressure is reduced (e.g., after hemorrhage), capillary diameter will be reduced even if alveolar pressure is normal.

Pulmonary Vascular Pressure–Flow Relationships

The *pressure–flow relationship* of a system can be measured by connecting it to a reservoir, as shown

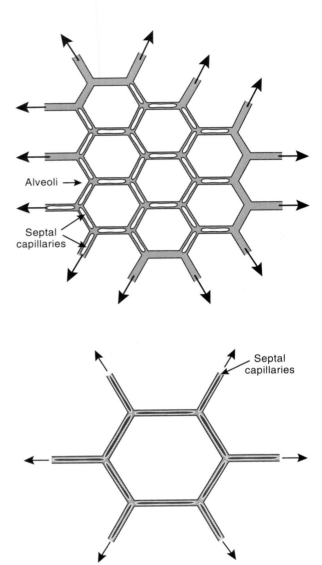

Figure 4–2. Septal capillaries at different lung volumes. Pulmonary alveolar septal capillaries reside in the septal walls of the alveoli. Since there is little structural reinforcement in the alveolar septa, the shape and volume of these capillaries are highly dependent on their transmural pressure (inside–outside pressure difference). Increases in alveolar volume tend to stretch and distort the capillaries, increasing their resistance to blood flow.

in Figure 4–3. If the reservoir is lifted slowly, the pressure driving flow through the system will rise. If the instantaneous flow rate is plotted against the driving pressure, a pressure–flow relationship is generated. Recall that for a straight tube the pressure–flow relationship will be linear, as long as the flow is laminar. This is equivalent to saying that

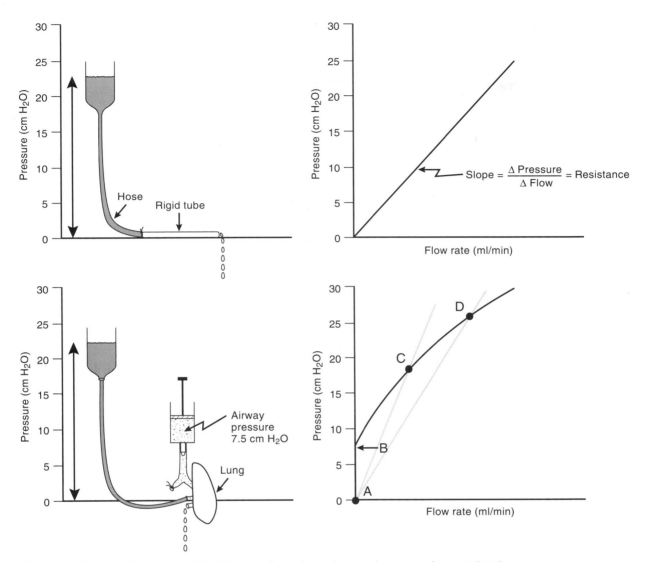

Figure 4–3. Pressure–flow relationships. Pressure–flow relationships can be measured in straight tubes (*upper*) or in the lung (*lower*) by connecting them to a reservoir that is lifted progressively to gradually increase the driving pressure, as instantaneous flow is measured. Under laminar flow conditions, the resulting pressure–flow relationship is linear for the straight tube but nonlinear for the lung. See text for further explanation.

the resistance of a straight tube is constant, since the slope of this straight line is the flow resistance (Figure 4–3). Since the pressure–flow relationship for the pulmonary circulation is nonlinear, its vascular resistance must change at different levels of flow. Consider what happens as the driving pressure is increased slowly across the lung. As shown in Figure 4–3, there is no flow in the system as the pressure rises from point A to B, so resistance must be infinite in that range. When the pressure exceeds that at point B, flow begins and increases as the driving pressure rises toward point C. Note that flow increases more for a given increment in pressure in the range C to D than in the range B to C. The slopes of the straight lines AC and AD are the vascular resistances at points C and D. By this analysis, the vascular resistance at point D is less than the resistance at C, even though nothing was done to vasodilate the vessels between those points. The important message from this analysis is that the relationship between pressure and flow in the pulmonary circulation is not linear; consequently any calculations of pulmonary vascular resistance will vary depending on the flow rate used.

Since the pulmonary arteries and veins contain relatively less smooth muscle in their walls than systemic vessels, they are more susceptible to mechanical distortion by high transmural pressures (i.e., they are more compliant) than their systemic counterparts. Since the distending pressure at point D is higher than at C, the pulmonary vessels are *distended* to a larger diameter, contributing to the lower resistance at point D. In addition, not all vascular channels in the pulmonary circulation are open at low pressures, so raising the intravascular pressure tends to open up additional pathways for

flow. This *vascular recruitment* also contributes to the fall in vascular resistance seen at higher transmural pressures. Because pulmonary vascular resistance changes passively in response to changes in vascular pressure, it is important to consider this influence when using pulmonary vascular resistance as a measure of active vasoconstriction in the pulmonary circulation.

Clinical Measurement of Pulmonary Vascular Pressures and Flows

Pressures in the pulmonary circulation are more difficult to measure than systemic blood pressure, since the pulmonary vessels are all within the chest. A procedure known as *right heart catheterization* can be used to measure pressures in the pulmonary circulation. One end of a fluid-filled tube (typically a 2- to 3-mm diameter catheter) is inserted into a systemic vein and advanced toward the heart. A special

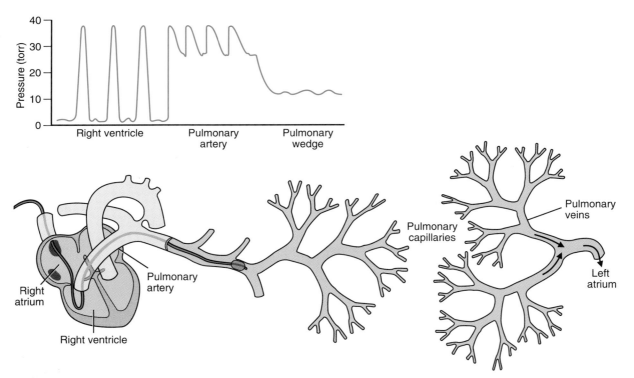

Figure 4-4. Measurement of pulmonary vascular pressures. During right heart catheterization, a fluid-filled catheter with a balloon near its tip is advanced from the vena cava through the right atrium and ventricle into the pulmonary artery. When the tip wedges into a branch of the pulmonary artery, blood flow beyond the balloon ceases and the pressure at the catheter tip (pulmonary wedge pressure) approximates left atrial pressure. Different pressures are recorded as the catheter tip passes through the heart into the pulmonary circulation.

balloon near the tip of the catheter is inflated with air, causing the tip of the catheter to be carried with the blood flow through the right atrium and into the right ventricle. The catheter is then advanced farther until the tip passes through the valve into the pulmonary artery. As the catheter tip moves through the chambers of the heart, different pressures are recorded from a pressure transducer connected to the external end of the catheter (Figure 4–4). When the catheter tip lodges in a branch of the pulmonary artery, it occludes blood flow in all of the downstream vessels supplied by that artery. Since those vessels still contain blood, a static column of blood is created from the distal tip of the catheter through the pulmonary capillaries to the point where the vein draining those vessels joins with other veins near the entrance to the left atrium. In this situation, the pressure measured at the tip of the catheter is the same throughout the static column of blood and is about the same as left atrial pressure. When air is let out of the balloon, flow

resumes in that branch of the pulmonary artery and the pressure at the tip again rises to the pulmonary artery pressure. The left atrial pressure measurement obtained by inflating the balloon around the tip of a catheter in the pulmonary artery is referred to as the *pulmonary capillary wedge pressure.*

Pulmonary blood flow (cardiac output) can be measured clinically using a technique known as *thermodilution.* Many of the catheters used for right heart catheterization are also equipped with a small, sensitive temperature sensor near the distal tip. To understand how this is useful for measurement of cardiac output, consider a system composed of a large reservoir (heated to 37°C) with a pump, as shown in Figure 4–5. The system pumps water from the reservoir through a long tube, which returns the water to the reservoir. A sensitive probe monitors the temperature near the outflow, and a syringe is used to inject ice-cold water upstream from the probe. Consider the situation when the pump is adjusted to a flow rate of 5 liters/min and

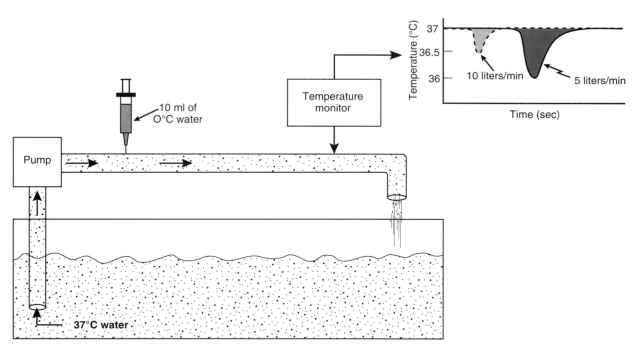

Figure 4–5. Measurement of pulmonary blood flow. Pulmonary blood flows can be measured using the principle of thermodilution. This technique is illustrated by considering a water-filled (37°C) reservoir equipped with a pump (analogous to the heart) and a long pipe (analogous to the pulmonary circulation). Water is pumped down the pipe at an adjustable flow rate. Boluses of 0°C water (10 ml) are injected upstream, and the transient temperature change is measured downstream. The area under the temperature–time curve is inversely proportional to the pump flow rate.

10 ml of ice water is injected into the flow. After a short delay, the temperature sensed near the outflow would decrease transiently as the bolus of cold water moved past it (Figure 4–5, *inset*). The speed of the pump is then decreased to 2.5 liters/min, and another 10 ml of ice water is injected. After a longer delay, the water temperature near the outflow would decrease by just as much as in the prior test but the bolus would spend twice as much time in contact with the temperature probe. Thus, the area under the temperature–time curve would be twice as large in the second case as the first. Based on the assumption that heat is neither lost nor gained from blood through the walls of the heart and the pulmonary artery, cardiac output can be measured in an analogous manner. Injections of cold solutions (usually 5% dextrose in water) are made into the right atrium while the temperature is measured by a sensor embedded in the side of the catheter in the pulmonary artery. From conservation of energy, the flow in the pulmonary artery can be calculated if the temperature–time curve is integrated (to determine the area) and if the volume and temperature of the injected bolus are known. Since this computation involves numerous calculations, small *cardiac output computers* are used to carry out the analysis.

Regional Pulmonary Blood Flows

Some regions of the lung normally receive more blood flow than others because of the effects of gravity on the pulmonary circulation. The blood flow that any particular region of lung receives depends on its *effective upstream and downstream pressures* and on the *caliber of the vessels* in the region. Gravity alters the distribution of regional blood flow by influencing each of these factors. Figure 4–6 shows the relative pulmonary blood flow as a function of distance from the bottom to the top of a vertical lung. Although there is a small decrease in relative blood flow at the very bottom of the lung, alveoli near the base of the lung tend to be much better perfused than alveoli near the top. Note that since the gradient in blood flow is a result of the effects of gravity, this relationship would be inverted if the subject were suspended upside down.

To understand the factors contributing to the regional differences in blood flow, consider what happens as blood enters the pulmonary circulation after leaving the right ventricle in an adult subject

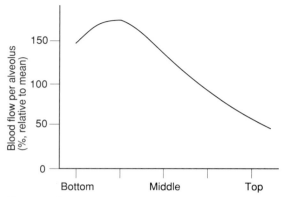

Figure 4–6. Regional differences in blood flow per alveolus. Gravity influences the regional blood flow from the top to the bottom of the lung at TLC. Although there is a small decrease in perfusion at the very bottom of the lung, alveoli near the bottom of the lung tend to be better perfused than alveoli near the top. (Redrawn from Hughes JMB, Glazier JB, Maloney JE, West JB: Effect of lung volume on the distribution of pulmonary blood flow in man. Respir Physiol 4:58–72, 1968.)

standing upright (Figure 4–7). Just outside the pulmonic valve, the main pulmonary artery hydrostatic pressure is about 18 torr. Blood going to the uppermost (apical) regions of the lung must travel vertically up the lung to reach the top. For every centimeter in height the blood rises, its hydrostatic pressure decreases by 1 cm H_2O (1 cm H_2O is equivalent to 0.74 torr). If the highest point in the lung is 15 cm above the pulmonic valve, the pulmonary artery pressure at the top of the lung will be 15 cm H_2O *less* than 18 torr, or about 6.9 torr. Conversely, blood traveling to lung regions below the heart will *increase* in pressure by 1 cm H_2O for every centimeter below the valve it reaches. Thus, a lung region 8 cm below the pulmonic valve would have a pulmonary arterial pressure of about 24 torr. Hence, *upstream* pressures in the pulmonary circulation can vary markedly from the upper to lower regions of the lung, owing to the influence of gravity.

Venous pressures in the pulmonary circulation also vary from the top to the bottom of a vertical lung for the same reason that arterial pressure varies. Under normal circumstances, left atrial pressure is about 5 torr. Thus, blood exiting from capillaries will exhibit venous pressures greater than left atrial pressure when the capillaries are located below the level of the left atrium and less than left

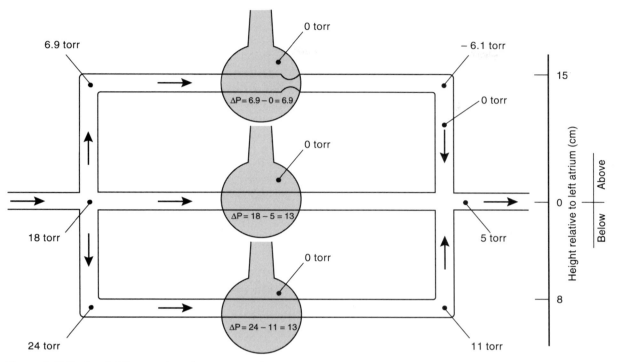

Figure 4–7. Regional differences in pulmonary vascular pressures. Regional pulmonary blood flow is determined by the effective upstream and downstream pressures and the caliber of the vessels. See text for further explanation. (Redrawn from Dawson CA, et al. Effects of lung inflation on longitudinal distribution of pulmonary vascular resistance. J Appl Physiol 43:1089–1092, 1977)

atrial pressure when they are situated above the level of the left atrium.

Local venous pressure is the *effective downstream pressure* only when it exceeds alveolar pressure. When the local venous pressure is less than alveolar pressure, the effective downstream pressure influencing flow becomes the alveolar pressure. Consider what happens when arterial pressure is greater than alveolar pressure, but alveolar pressure is greater than venous pressure. In this condition, the venous end of the capillary tends to collapse because of its negative transmural pressure. Yet if this occurred, flow in the capillary would cease and cause the intravascular pressure at the venous end to rise toward arterial pressure. This would reopen the capillary and restore flow causing the capillary to collapse again. In the end, alveolar septal capillaries in this state remain open along their length but become narrowed near the venous end. Note that blood flow in these capillaries is determined by the difference between arterial and alveolar pressures and is independent of changes in the venous pressure as long as the venous pressure remains less than the alveolar pressure. By analogy, the flow of a river over a waterfall is independent of the height of the waterfall because the flow is controlled by factors upstream of the waterfall. This analogy has led to the term *vascular waterfall* to describe the factors influencing vascular flow under conditions in which venous pressure is less than alveolar pressure.

EXAMPLE. Main pulmonary arterial pressure is 18 torr, and left atrial pressure is 5 torr. Calculate the *effective* upstream and downstream pressures for an alveolus at 7 cm above and 5 cm below the level of the left atrium in a lung where the alveolar pressure is 2 cm H_2O.

At the level of the left atrium, the effective upstream pressure is 18 torr and venous pressure is 5 torr. Because venous pressure is greater than alveolar pressure, the effective downstream pressure is 5 torr. In the alveolus 5 cm below the left atrium, effective upstream pressure is 21.7 torr (18 torr + 5 cm · 0.74 torr/cm H_2O). Venous pressure is 8.7 torr (5 torr + 5 cm · 0.74 torr/cm H_2O) and is the effective downstream pressure, because it is greater than alveolar pressure. For an alveolus 7 cm above the left atrium, effective upstream pressure is 12.8 torr (18 torr − 7 cm · 0.74 torr/cm H_2O). Because venous pressure (+ 1.3 torr = 5 torr − 5 cm · 0.74 torr/cm H_2O) is less than alveolar pressure, the effective downstream pressure is alveolar pressure (2 cm H_2O or 1.5 torr). ■

Zones of the Lung

Based on the local factors influencing blood flow (i.e., upstream, downstream, and alveolar pressures), different regions of the lung can be classified into three functional zones (Figure 4–8). In zone I regions, alveolar pressure is greater than the local pulmonary arterial or venous pressures. Because the

alveolar pressure exceeds the intravascular pressure, the capillaries within the alveolar walls are pressed shut and no flow occurs in them. Zone I conditions are most likely to occur at the top of the lung, since intravascular pressures are lowest at that point. Although zone I conditions do not normally exist in a healthy subject, they can develop if alveolar pressure is increased during positive-pressure ventilation or if pulmonary artery pressure is reduced (as during hemorrhage). In zone III regions, the local pulmonary arterial pressure is greater than the venous pressure, and both are greater than the alveolar pressure. In this condition, alveolar capillary flow is set by the arteriovenous pressure difference and the caliber of the blood vessels. Under normal conditions, alveoli near the bottom of a lung are most likely to operate under zone III conditions. However, when a subject lies down, the maximum vertical distance from the top to the bottom of the lung is reduced and more of it operates under zone III conditions. In zone II, pulmonary arterial pressure is greater than either alveolar or venous pressure, so flow occurs. Since alveolar pressure exceeds venous pressure, a vascular waterfall condition exists, and local flow is determined by the arterial-alveolar pressure difference. Normally, the top third of a vertical lung operates in zone II conditions.

Effects of Lung Volume on Vascular Resistance

As lung volume changes, the transmural forces acting on the pulmonary circulation also change, causing blood vessels to vary in caliber and shape. This changes the pulmonary vascular resistance in the manner shown in Figure 4–9. At functional residual capacity (FRC), overall vascular resistance is at its lowest point. As lung volume increases above FRC, the resistance to blood flow increases, reaching its highest point at total lung capacity (TLC). This increase in resistance is due primarily to the increase in alveolar volume, which stretches and distorts capillaries in the alveolar septal walls. This is analogous to the way that pulling on opposite edges of a floppy plastic bag tends to narrow its diameter (see Figure 4–2, lower). The greater the reduction in capillary diameter, the greater the increase in resistance. When lung volume is reduced below FRC, vascular resistance also tends to increase. This effect is mainly due to an increase in the

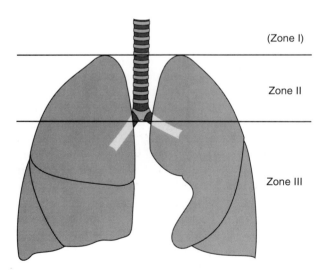

(Zone I)

Zone II

Zone III

Figure 4–8. Zones of the lung. Because of the effects of gravity on the effective upstream and downstream pressures, different lung regions operate under different flow conditions. Most of the normal lung operates under zone III conditions, which tend to occur in lower regions of the lung. Some of the lung operates under zone II conditions, toward the top of the lung. Although zone I conditions do not normally occur, they are most likely to develop in the uppermost regions of the lung.

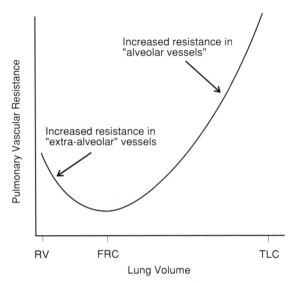

Figure 4-9. Pulmonary vascular resistance as a function of lung volume. Pulmonary vascular resistance is lowest near functional residual capacity. Increases at higher lung volumes are caused by the increase in resistance in alveolar vessels. The increase in resistance below functional residual capacity is due to the increased resistance in extra-alveolar vessels.

vessels supplying those alveoli that are hypoxic and that it is more vigorous at lower alveolar oxygen tensions.

The effects of hypoxic pulmonary vasoconstriction depend on how many alveoli have reduced P_{O_2} (hypoxia) and how low the alveolar P_{O_2} is. For example, if a subject travels to high altitude where the barometric pressure is reduced, inspired P_{O_2} will decrease, and the alveolar P_{O_2} will be reduced in every alveolus. Under this situation, vasoconstriction will occur in all precapillary vessels, causing an increase in mean pulmonary arterial pressure but little change in the regional distribution of pulmonary blood flow. On the other hand, if the alveolar P_{O_2} is selectively reduced in only some alveoli, the local vasoconstriction will shift blood flow away from those hypoxic regions toward alveoli with normal P_{O_2} *(normoxic)*. In this sense, hypoxic pulmonary vasoconstriction may help to improve lung gas exchange by reducing blood flow in alveoli with abnormally low alveolar P_{O_2}. For example, if a lung lobe were to collapse or become filled with edema fluid, its alveolar P_{O_2} would decrease (because its

resistance of the larger vessels upstream and downstream from the alveolar vessels. When lung volume is at or above FRC, these *extra-alveolar vessels* tend to be stretched open by their connections with alveoli and connective tissue (Figure 4–10). This *tethering* tends to augment their diameter, thereby minimizing their resistance. When lung volume is below FRC, the tethering effect is less, and the caliber of the alveolar vessels is reduced, causing their resistance to increase. At low lung volumes, the resistance in alveolar vessels is less.

HYPOXIC PULMONARY VASOCONSTRICTION

Hypoxic pulmonary vasoconstriction is an active constriction of vascular smooth muscle in pulmonary vessels upstream from the capillaries that occurs when the P_{O_2} of alveolar gas is reduced. The response is intrinsic to the lung, thus it can also occur in transplanted or excised lungs. Although it has been the focus of a large amount of study, the mechanism underlying the hypoxic pulmonary vasoconstrictor response is still not known. What is known is that the vasoconstriction only occurs in

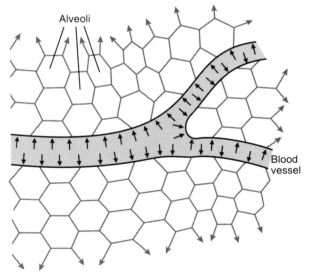

Figure 4-10. Extra-alveolar blood vessels. Extra-alveolar blood vessels are those that are not directly influenced by changes in alveolar pressure. The caliber of extra-alveolar blood vessels changes with lung volume because the vessel wall is tethered by its connections with surrounding alveoli. At low lung volumes the traction provided by surrounding tissue is reduced, thereby increasing the resistance to blood flow.

$\dot{V}A/\dot{Q}$ ratio has decreased—see Chapter 7). Hypoxic pulmonary vasoconstriction in the unventilated lobe diverts blood flow toward better ventilated lung regions. In normal lungs, small amounts of hypoxic vasoconstriction contribute to the matching of ventilation–perfusion ratios by adjusting local alveolar blood flows in accord with local alveolar oxygen tensions.

LUNG FLUID BALANCE

Factors Influencing Fluid Movement Across the Pulmonary Vascular Wall

The pulmonary circulation has an enormous surface area. Because the sum of the forces tending to move liquid out of the circulation into the interstitial space slightly exceeds the forces tending to hold fluid in, there is a continuous flux of fluid from the vascular space into the interstitium. Most of this fluid is removed from the lung by the *pulmonary lymphatic system,* which channels the fluid through a series of ducts and lymph nodes to eventually drain into the vena cava.

Figure 4–11 summarizes the balance of forces tending to promote *fluid filtration* out of the vessels versus those promoting *fluid reabsorption. Hydrostatic pressure differences* between the vascular and interstitial compartments normally move fluids out of the vessels across the semipermeable barrier presented by the blood vessel wall. Because the permeability of the pulmonary vessels to proteins is small, the protein concentration in the plasma is greater than in the interstitium. This causes an *oncotic pressure difference* across the vessel wall, which normally acts to draw water osmotically from the interstitial space into the vascular compartment. The relative magnitudes of the hydrostatic and oncotic pressures between the blood plasma (intravascular) and the surrounding extravascular space (interstitium) determine the direction and flow rate of the fluid *(flux)* into or out of the vessels. Since most of the surface area available for fluid exchange is in the capillaries, most analyses of lung fluid balance focus on these vessels, even though larger vessels can also exchange fluid with the interstitium.

In the pulmonary circulation, the hydrostatic pressure within the capillaries is less than arterial but greater than venous pressure. Since about 60%

of the total resistance to pulmonary blood flow resides in the vessels upstream of the capillaries, average capillary pressure can be estimated by subtracting 60% of the arteriovenous pressure difference from the pulmonary arterial pressure. For example, if arterial pressure is 18 torr and left atrial pressure is 5 torr, capillary hydrostatic pressure will be about 10 torr. Interstitial hydrostatic pressure is difficult to determine directly, and experimental attempts to measure it have yielded widely differing values. However, most studies indicate that interstitial pressure is negative by about 12 torr. Intravascular and interstitial colloid osmotic pressures can be estimated from measurements of plasma and lymphatic fluid using a membrane oncometer. Studies suggest that interstitial colloid osmotic pressure is normally about 10 torr, when plasma colloidal pressure is 20 torr.

Using the above values, the lung transvascular fluid flux can be calculated using the *Starling equation:*

$$\text{Flux} = K_{fc}[(Piv - Pis) - \sigma_d(\pi iv - \pi is)]$$

The calculated flux has units of flow (ml/min). The term K_{fc} is called the *capillary filtration coefficient* and has units of conductance (1/resistance). This value depends heavily on the total number of capillaries that are perfused and is difficult to quantify. The terms Piv and Pis are the hydrostatic pressures in the intravascular (iv) and interstitial (is) compartments, while πiv and πis refer to the intravascular and interstitial colloid osmotic pressures, respectively. The term σ_d is termed the *reflection coefficient.* The reflection coefficient is a measure of how permeable the membrane is to the proteins exerting the oncotic pressure. When σ_d is 1.0, the membrane is impermeable to the proteins, and any change in protein concentration on one side of the membrane will exert its full osmotic effect. On the other hand, if proteins can pass easily through the membrane, a change in protein concentration on one side will have little oncotic effect, and σ_d will approach zero. When σ_d is small, the net fluid flux is determined mainly by the hydrostatic pressure difference. Normally, σ_d averages about 0.75. Note that the net fluid flux reflects a balance between the forces tending to force fluid out (Piv and πis) and the forces tending to force fluid in (Pis and πiv). When the flux is positive, the forces tending to drive fluid out of

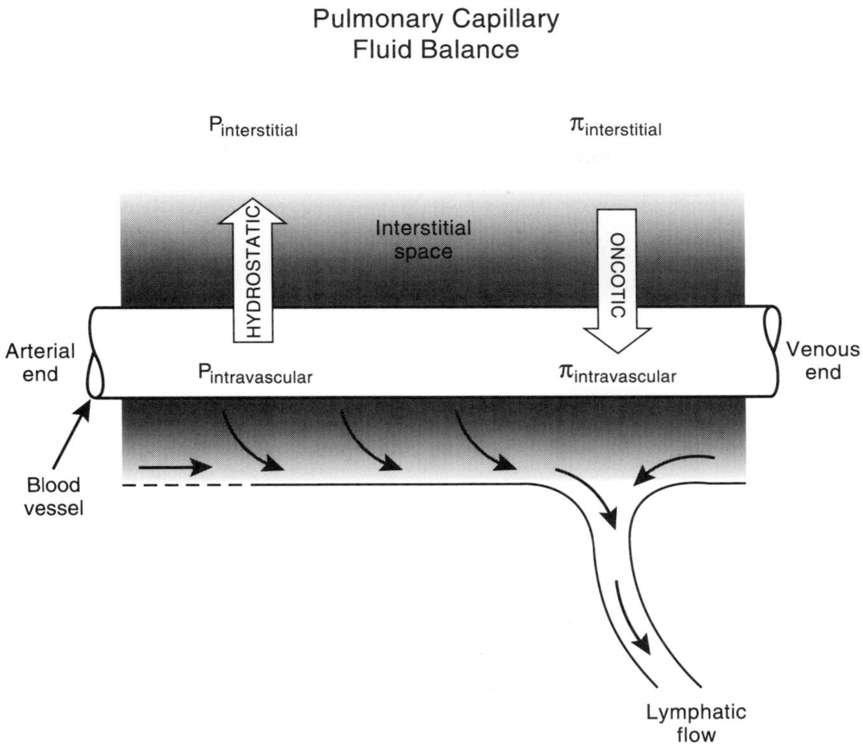

Pulmonary Capillary
Fluid Balance

Figure 4–11. Factors influencing lung fluid balance. The Starling equation summarizes the balance of forces favoring fluid flux into or out of the pulmonary vessels. Normally there is a net flux of fluid out of the vessels, which is drained from the interstitial space by the lymphatic system.

the capillary predominate, whereas a negative flux indicates that net fluid reabsorption is favored.

Applying the Starling equation to the above values of hydrostatic and oncotic pressures yields a positive value, indicating that there will be a net filtration of fluid out of the capillary:

$$\text{Flux} = K_{fc}\{[10 - (-12)] - 0.75(10)\}$$

$$\text{Flux} = K_{fc}(22 - 7.5)$$

From a practical standpoint, the Starling equation is not especially useful because measurements of interstitial pressure and oncotic pressure are imprecise. Moreover, the value of K_{fc} depends on the surface area available for filtration, and it varies depending on the number of capillaries in the lung that are recruited. The reflection coefficient σ_d varies with the size of protein molecule being examined and cannot be measured except under highly controlled experimental conditions. Finally, capil-

lary hydrostatic pressures vary widely from the top to the bottom of the lung so this equation applies only to a given level in the lung.

The Pulmonary Lymphatic System

The Starling equation summarizes the balance between forces tending to drive water out of the pulmonary circulation and those tending to retain water in the vascular space. Normally, the small flux of fluid out of the vascular compartment enters the interstitium surrounding the capillaries. From there it travels to the alveolar corners and then to the peribronchial interstitial space surrounding the bronchi and small arteries. From this point, the fluid enters the lymphatic system and travels through the interstitial space to exit from the lung at the hilum. Estimates suggest that the lung lymphatics normally return 10 to 50 ml fluid/hr to the systemic circulation in an adult human. If the rate of fluid filtration is increased moderately, the rate of lymphatic clearance also increases.

Pulmonary Edema

When the rate of fluid filtration out of the capillaries exceeds the ability of the lymphatics to remove it, fluid begins to accumulate in the interstitial spaces of the lung. As fluid accumulates, the pressure in the interstitium rises and the lymphatic vessels swell in size. This condition is termed *interstitial edema,* and it does not interfere significantly with gas exchange because the alveoli remain open and continue to exchange gas normally. However, when interstitial fluid pressure increases above a certain point, fluid leaks through the alveolar epithelium into the alveoli, where it accumulates. This condition, known as *alveolar edema,* can dramatically interfere with lung gas exchange. After a small amount of edema enters an alveolus, the effects of surface tension cause the alveolus to shrink in volume until the edema completely fills it. Histological samples from lungs with alveolar edema typically show some alveoli that are gas filled and of normal size and others that are small and completely filled with edema fluid. Since capillary blood flow continues even when an alveolus is filled with edema, no gas exchange occurs along these capillaries. Hence, alveolar edema is associated with the development of significant *shunting,* which can lead to systemic *arterial hypoxemia* (see Chapter 7).

Pulmonary edema is classified according to the cause of the increased fluid filtration. In *hydrostatic* or *high pressure pulmonary edema,* the edema forms because the hydrostatic pressure in the pulmonary capillaries is abnormally increased. Clinically, this can occur in left-ventricular heart failure, when increases in left atrial pressure cause the pulmonary venous (and thus capillary) pressures to increase. Hydrostatic edema often resolves rapidly (within hours) after the pressures return to normal, as the lymphatic clearance catches up with the rate of fluid filtration.

The other type of lung edema is termed *low pressure* or *high permeability edema.* The hydrostatic pressures are normal in this form of edema, but the permeability of the capillary endothelium to protein is increased. In the Starling equation, this is seen as a decrease in the reflection coefficient (σ_d). Permeability can be increased when the endothelium is damaged by hyperoxia, drugs, chemicals, bacterial endotoxins, transiently high pressures, or inflammatory mediators. Neutrophils that adhere to the pulmonary capillaries and release toxic oxygen radicals (see Chapter 11) are also thought to damage the endothelial cells and may contribute to the development of edema in certain disease states. To distinguish between high permeability and high pressures as the cause of pulmonary edema, it is usually necessary to measure the pressures in the pulmonary circulation using right heart catheterization. If pressures are not abnormally elevated, increased permeability is generally suspected as the cause. In some circumstances a sample of alveolar fluid can be obtained for analysis of protein content. When the alveolar fluid protein concentration is much lower than in plasma, high pressure edema is suspected.

Clearance of Pulmonary Edema

When the cause of the increased fluid filtration is removed, edematous lungs gradually remove the excess fluid in a process of *edema clearance.* Most edema is cleared by the lymphatic drainage, although some fluid may be reabsorbed into the pulmonary circulation or it may enter the pleural space. Most alveolar edema is cleared by ion pumps in alveolar epithelial cells, which transport ions from alveolar fluid into the interstitium. As this process occurs, water is drawn osmotically through the epithelium into the interstitial space, where it can enter the lymphatic system.

Chapter 5

Oxygen and Carbon Dioxide Transport in Blood

The cells of the body carry out a variety of metabolic functions, including some that are essential to maintain cell integrity and others that allow cells to function collectively as tissues and organs. The former category includes processes such as active ion pumping and cell growth and repair, while the latter includes contraction, membrane transport, biosynthesis, and other metabolic processes. These active cell processes require energy expenditure. In most cells these energetic demands are met by oxidative metabolism, which produces adenosine triphosphate (ATP) in the mitochondrial electron transport system as molecular oxygen is consumed.

Under resting conditions, the concentration of oxygen within the mitochondria is normally far greater than required to support electron transport. Consequently, the rate of ATP formation is set by metabolic demand rather than by the local availability of oxygen. The cardiopulmonary system functions to maintain this state by transporting enough oxygen from the lungs to the cells of the body to maintain tissue metabolic activity while carrying carbon dioxide back to the lungs for elimination. In this chapter, the focus is on the mechanisms involved in the carriage of oxygen and carbon dioxide in blood and on the factors that influence the uptake and release of these gases as blood passes through the capillaries of the lung and the systemic tissues. An important concept developed in this chapter is the interdependency of the simultaneous oxygen and carbon dioxide transport in blood. In this regard, the uptake of oxygen into blood passing through the pulmonary capillaries is facilitated by the simultaneous release of carbon dioxide from the blood into alveolar gas. Likewise, the release of carbon dioxide is facilitated by the simultaneous uptake of oxygen. In this sense, blood is ideally suited to the simultaneous transport of oxygen to the tissues and the transport of carbon dioxide to the lungs.

Systemic Oxygen Delivery and Consumption: The Fick Relationship

The cardiac output ($\dot{Q}t$) is defined as the volume of blood pumped by the heart to the systemic tissues each minute (Figure 5–1). As blood passes through the systemic capillaries, some of the oxygen it carries leaves the capillaries and enters the tissue;

the remainder of the oxygen stays in the blood and returns to the heart and lungs. The total volume of oxygen transported to the systemic tissues per minute (*systemic oxygen delivery*) is the product of the $\dot{Q}t$ and the oxygen content of arterial blood:

$$\text{Systemic oxygen delivery} =$$

$$\dot{Q}t \cdot \text{arterial blood oxygen content}$$

The unused volume of oxygen that returns from the systemic tissues per minute is the product of the cardiac output and the mixed venous blood oxygen content:

$$\text{Oxygen returning} =$$

$$\dot{Q}t \cdot \text{mixed venous blood oxygen content}$$

Hence, the rate of oxygen consumption by systemic tissues ($\dot{V}_{O_2}$) must equal the difference between the rates of oxygen delivery and oxygen returning:

$$\dot{V}_{O_2} = \dot{Q}t \cdot (Ca_{O_2} - C\bar{v}_{O_2})$$

where Ca_{O_2} and $C\bar{v}_{O_2}$ are the oxygen contents of arterial and mixed venous blood, respectively. This is the *Fick relationship*, which is based on the principle of conservation of mass. Oxygen content in blood is usually expressed in units of milliliters of oxygen per deciliter of blood (abbreviated as ml/dl) or equivalently as volume percent (vol%). Note that the units of oxygen content in blood are identical to units of concentration.

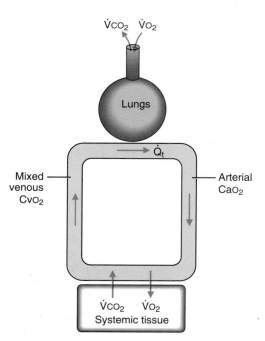

EXAMPLE. A subject has a cardiac output of 5 liters/min, an arterial blood oxygen content of 19 ml/dl, and a mixed venous blood oxygen content of 14 ml/dl. What is the systemic oxygen consumption?

Using the above relationship,

$$\dot{V}_{O_2} = (50 \text{ dl/min})(19 \text{ ml/dl} - 14 \text{ ml/dl})$$

$$= 250 \text{ ml/min.} \quad \blacksquare$$

Figure 5–1. The Fick relationship for oxygen transport. Systemic oxygen delivery (ml/min) is the product of the cardiac output ($\dot{Q}t$, dl/min) and the content of oxygen in arterial blood (Ca_{O_2}, ml/dl). The rate at which unused oxygen is delivered back to the heart (returning O_2, ml/min) is calculated as the product of $\dot{Q}t$ and the mixed venous blood oxygen content ($C\bar{v}_{O_2}$, ml/dl). The difference between these is the rate of systemic oxygen consumption ($\dot{V}_{O_2}$).

OXYGEN TRANSPORT IN BLOOD

Blood is composed of red blood cells (erythrocytes), white blood cells (leukocytes), and platelets suspended in plasma, a protein- and lipid-containing liquid. The percentage of the blood volume composed of red blood cells is referred to as the *hematocrit*. Normally, this value is 37% to 42% in premenopausal women and slightly higher in men. Red blood cells contain quantities of *hemoglobin,* a molecule specialized for the transport of oxygen and carbon dioxide. Since each red blood cell contains approximately the same amount of hemoglobin, the overall hemoglobin concentration in blood is proportional to the blood hematocrit. Oxygen is carried in two forms by blood. Most of the oxygen carried is bound to hemoglobin, whereas a smaller portion of the oxygen is physically dissolved in the blood.

Oxygen Transport by Hemoglobin

Hemoglobin is a molecule composed of four polypeptide chains *(globin)*, each of which is linked to an iron-containing porphyrin ring *(heme)*. The heme groups give rise to the characteristic red color of blood. Red blood cells formed during intrauterine development contain a fetal form of hemoglobin *(hemoglobin f)* composed of two α polypeptide chains (141 amino acids each) and two γ polypeptide chains (146 amino acids). (see Chapter 10.) After birth, newly formed red blood cells contain adult hemoglobin *(hemoglobin A)*; these gradually replace the cells containing hemoglobin f. Hemoglobin A is also a tetramer, composed of two α and two β chains (146 amino acids) that share some similarities with the γ chains. These polypeptide chains mesh closely and are held together by hydrogen bonds and hydrophobic attractions. In its normal conformation, the interior of the hemoglobin molecule is highly hydrophobic while the exterior is hydrophilic. Because one oxygen molecule can reversibly bind to each heme group, a maximum of four oxygen molecules can be carried by a single hemoglobin molecule (Figure 5–2). The heme groups are situated within hydrophobic crevices in the globin molecule, and each contains an iron atom oxidized to the ferrous (2 +) state. This hydrophobic environment protects the iron ion from being oxidized to the ferric (3 +) state by water. Since molecular oxygen is lipophilic, it can gain access easily to the hydrophobic environment of the heme group where it binds reversibly. The optical absorption spectrum of hemoglobin shifts when oxygen binds to a heme group, which causes the difference in color between oxygenated and deoxygenated hemoglobin forms.

When oxygen combines with hemoglobin, the iron atom normally remains in the ferrous state. However, compounds such as ferricyanide (as well as certain drugs) can oxidize the iron to the ferric state and cause a change in the color of hemoglobin from red to brown. The resulting compound *(methemoglobin)* cannot function as a reversible oxygen carrier. *Glutathione reductase enzymes* present in red blood cells have the ability to reduce methemoglobin to hemoglobin, thereby restoring its ability to function as an oxygen carrier. Normally, 1% to 2% of the binding sites in blood are oxidized to the ferric state at any time.

The avidity with which oxygen binds to hemoglobin is heavily influenced by the tertiary structure of the hemoglobin molecule and the changes in confirmation that it undergoes as oxygen is bound or released. A genetic alteration resulting in a single amino acid substitution in one of the chains may produce a dramatic change in the binding affinity of hemoglobin for oxygen. Genetic alterations that produce amino acid substitutions at critical locations in the protein may prove fatal because they render the molecule ineffective as a reversible carrier of oxygen. However, a large number of naturally occurring genetic alterations have been identified, many of which cause moderate alterations in the oxygen binding or other characteristics of the molecule. For example, in sickle cell anemia a valine amino acid replaces a glutamic acid residue on the β chain. This single amino acid substitution promotes the protein to form a gel in its deoxygenated state. When the hemoglobin forms a gel, the red blood cells distort from their normal biconcave disk shape into a crescent-like shape. Sickled cells are liable to form thrombi, resulting in a sickle cell crisis.

Dissolved Oxygen in Blood

Part of the oxygen carried in blood remains physically dissolved in the lipid and aqueous components of the blood. Figure 5–3 shows the relationship between the concentration of dissolved oxygen and

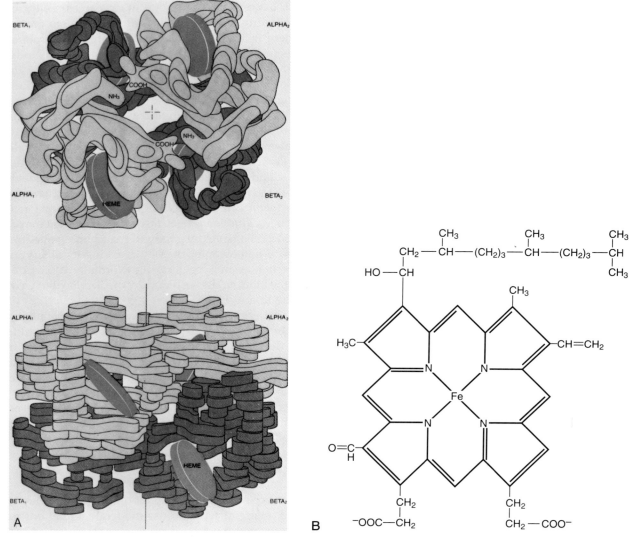

Figure 5-2. The hemoglobin molecule. *A.* Oxygen binds reversibly at four porphyrin (heme) groups on the hemoglobin molecule. The heme groups are situated within hydrophobic nooks in the globin portion, making the ferrous (2^+) ion accessible to lipophilic molecules such as oxygen and carbon monoxide but largely inaccessible to water. (*A*, redrawn from Perutz MF: Sci Am 239:68–83, 1978. Copyright © 1978, by Scientific American, Inc., George V. Kelvin, all rights reserved.) *B.* Chemical structure of the porphyrin (heme) groups, showing the ferrous ion where oxygen binds reversibly.

the *partial pressure of oxygen in blood.* The partial pressure of a gas in a liquid is somewhat analogous to a hydrostatic pressure of a fluid in a pipe (or a voltage in an electrical conductor), in the sense that it represents a potential force that will determine how vigorously the gas will try to leave the liquid. The partial pressures of gases in blood are impor-

tant, for they determine the direction and velocity at which the gases diffuse into or out of the blood as it passes through a capillary. One could adjust the P_{O_2} in blood by exposing a volume of blood to a gas mixture with the desired P_{O_2} and allowing the two to come to equilibrium (Figure 5-4). However, since the *solubility* of oxygen in plasma is relatively

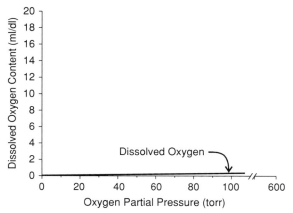

Figure 5-3. Dissolved oxygen content in blood. The relationship between the volume of oxygen dissolved in a liquid (ml/dl) and the partial pressure (tension) of oxygen in the liquid is linear. Hence, doubling the partial pressure will double the dissolved oxygen content. Symbol illustrates the dissolved oxygen content that would exist at a P_{O_2} of 600 torr.

low, the concentration of dissolved oxygen is smaller than the portion bound to hemoglobin (see later). Nevertheless, the dissolved oxygen component is still significant and should always be taken into consideration when considering blood oxygen content. The dissolved portion is proportional to the

P_{O_2} and is calculated by multiplying the oxygen tension (torr) by the oxygen solubility in plasma (0.00304 ml O_2/(dl · torr)).

Oxyhemoglobin Saturation and Blood Oxygen Content

The molecular weight of hemoglobin is approximately 64,500 daltons, and each molecule has the potential to bind four oxygen atoms. Thus, 1 mmol of hemoglobin (64.5 g) can carry up to 4 mmol of oxygen (4 × 22.4 ml/mmol = 89.6 ml/mmol) if all of the binding sites are occupied (i.e., when the hemoglobin is *fully saturated*). Hence, each gram of hemoglobin can theoretically bind 1.39 ml of oxygen when the saturation is 100%. The value of 1.39 ml/g is therefore referred to as the *theoretical oxygen binding capacity* of hemoglobin. In practice, about 4% of the binding sites cannot function as oxygen carriers because some of the hemoglobin is present as methemoglobin (1% to 2%) and some of the binding sites are occupied by carbon monoxide (1% to 2%). For this reason, a value of 1.34 ml/g is sometimes used instead of 1.39 to represent the *physiological oxygen binding capacity.*

The number of oxygen molecules bound to hemoglobin depends on the P_{O_2} in the blood. The

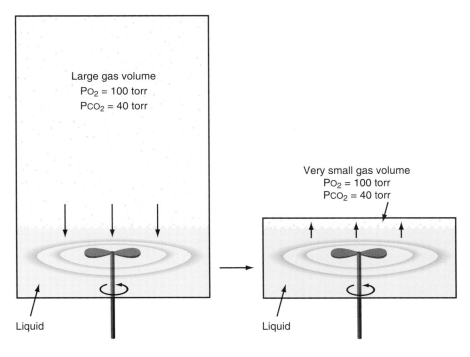

Figure 5-4. Gas partial pressure in a liquid. The P_{O_2} in blood is the oxygen tension that is in equilibrium with the dissolved oxygen. If a reservoir of gas with known oxygen tension is allowed to equilibrate with a volume of blood, oxygen will continue to enter the blood until the partial pressures in blood and gas are equal. If the gas reservoir is then replaced by a small gas volume that contains no oxygen, O_2 will diffuse from the blood into the new gas until the partial pressures in blood and gas are equal.

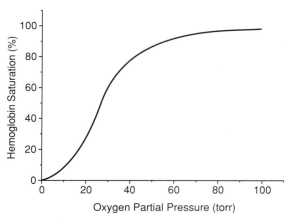

Figure 5–5. Oxyhemoglobin dissociation curve showing the relationship between the oxygen partial pressure in blood (Po_2) and the percentage of the hemoglobin binding sites that are occupied by oxygen molecules (percent saturation). Adult hemoglobin (hemoglobin A) is about 50% saturated at a Po_2 of 27 torr, 90% saturated at 60 torr, and about 98% saturated at 100 torr.

curve in Figure 5–5 shows the relationship between the Po_2 in blood and the percentage of the oxygen binding sites that are occupied by oxygen molecules *(hemoglobin percent saturation)*. If blood is equilibrated with a gas that contains no oxygen, then the hemoglobin saturation will decrease to zero because oxygen will have left all of the hemoglobin binding sites. Under normal conditions, blood equilibrated to a partial pressure of 27 torr will have about half of the binding sites occupied, while blood equilibrated to more than 150 torr will have essentially 100% of the binding sites occupied.

The hemoglobin molecule undergoes a conformational change as oxygen molecules bind or release, giving rise to the curvilinear shape of the oxyhemoglobin dissociation curve. When the first oxygen molecule leaves a fully oxygenated hemoglobin, the hemoglobin molecule undergoes a conformational change that allows the second and third oxygen molecules to release more easily. Conversely, binding of the first oxygen molecule onto a fully deoxygenated hemoglobin facilitates the binding of the second and third oxygen molecules. This alteration in binding affinity is manifested by a steeper change in saturation for a given change in Po_2 in the middle of the dissociation curve than at the extreme ends. The curvilinear relationship be-

tween Po_2 and percent saturation is well suited for the transport of oxygen from the lungs to the tissues.

Physiological Consequences of the Hemoglobin Dissociation Curve Shape

In a healthy subject at sea level, arterial blood normally has a Po_2 of about 95 torr, corresponding to about 97% hemoglobin saturation. Note that even if the Po_2 of blood leaving the lungs is reduced by as much as 20 to 30 torr (because of lung disease or high altitude), the arterial blood hemoglobin will still be nearly fully saturated, since the slope of the dissociation curve is relatively shallow in that range (Figure 5–5). Thus, the shape of the oxyhemoglobin dissociation curve "protects" the level of arterial saturation despite moderate reductions in the arterial Po_2.

As a red blood cell enters a systemic capillary, the Po_2 in the tissue surrounding the capillary is lower than in the blood and oxygen diffuses out of the capillary into the tissue. As oxygen diffuses out of the capillary, the Po_2 in the plasma surrounding the red blood cells falls. This causes oxygen to dissociate from hemoglobin inside the red blood cells and diffuse into the plasma. Oxygen continues to diffuse out as the blood moves through the capillary, and the hemoglobin saturation falls as progressively more oxygen is released. By the time the red blood cell exits from the end of the capillary, it will have released only a portion of the oxygen it carried. Under resting conditions, blood typically releases about 25% of its oxygen content along capillaries (average venous oxygen saturation = 75%), although the level of venous oxygen saturation varies widely among different tissues. During exercise, muscle tissue Po_2 decreases significantly as the myocytes consume oxygen, thereby augmenting the driving gradient for diffusion out of the capillaries. This allows muscles to extract more than 90% of the oxygen from blood during periods of heavy exercise.

Oxygen Content in Blood

The content of oxygen in blood represents the volume of oxygen contained per unit volume of blood and is usually referred to as the total *oxygen content.*

Although most of the oxygen contained in blood is bound to hemoglobin, the total oxygen content of blood is the sum of the hemoglobin-bound and the dissolved portions. The hemoglobin-bound portion of the oxygen content depends on the concentration of hemoglobin present (in g/dl), the oxygen binding capacity of the hemoglobin (1.39 ml O_2/g Hb), and the hemoglobin percent saturation. This point is best illustrated by a calculation of the oxygen content in a sample of blood.

EXAMPLE. A sample of arterial blood is obtained from a patient. Analysis reveals the following: Po_2 = 95 torr, hemoglobin concentration = 14 g/dl, hemoglobin saturation = 97%. Calculate the oxygen content as the sum of the dissolved and hemoglobin-bound components:

Dissolved oxygen content = Po_2(torr) · Solubility

$$\text{in} \left(\frac{\text{ml } O_2}{\text{dl} \cdot \text{torr}}\right) = 95 \cdot 0.00304 = 0.29 \left(\frac{\text{ml}}{\text{dl}}\right)$$

Hemoglobin-bound oxygen content =

$$1.39 \frac{\text{ml}}{\text{g Hb}} \cdot 14 \frac{\text{g Hb}}{\text{dl blood}} \cdot 0.97 \left(\frac{\% \text{ saturation}}{100}\right) =$$

$$18.88 \frac{\text{ml}}{\text{dl}}$$

Thus, the total oxygen content of the blood = $0.29 + 18.88 = 19.17 \frac{\text{ml}}{\text{dl}}$. ■

EXAMPLE. A sample of mixed venous blood is obtained from a patient by way of a catheter whose tip is positioned in the pulmonary artery. Analysis reveals the following: Po_2 = 40 torr, hemoglobin concentration = 14 g/dl, hemoglobin saturation = 74%. Calculate the oxygen content as the sum of the dissolved and hemoglobin-bound components:

Dissolved oxygen content = Po_2(torr) · Solubility

$$\text{in} \left(\frac{\text{ml } O_2}{\text{dl} \cdot \text{torr}}\right) = 40 \cdot 0.00304 = 0.12 \left(\frac{\text{ml}}{\text{dl}}\right)$$

Hemoglobin-bound oxygen content =

$$1.39 \frac{\text{ml}}{\text{g Hb}} \cdot 14 \frac{\text{g Hb}}{\text{dl blood}} \cdot 0.74 \left(\frac{\% \text{ saturation}}{100}\right) =$$

$$14.40 \frac{\text{ml}}{\text{dl}}$$

Thus, the total oxygen content of the blood = $0.12 + 14.40 = 14.52 \frac{\text{ml}}{\text{dl}}$. ■

Figure 5–6 shows the total oxygen content of blood as a function of Po_2, i.e., as the sum of hemoglobin-bound and dissolved components. Note that the dissolved oxygen portion represents less than 2% of the oxygen content in arterial blood. If the arterial Po_2 is increased to 600 torr by breathing 100% oxygen, the dissolved oxygen concentration will increase to about 1.8 ml/dl, or about 10% of the oxygen content in arterial blood. Since hemoglobin is fully oxygenated when the arterial Po_2 increases above about 150 torr, increasing the Po_2 further to 600 torr produces only a minor increment in arterial content.

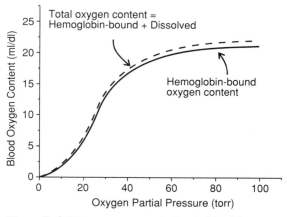

Figure 5–6. The oxygen concentration in blood (oxygen content) as the sum of the dissolved oxygen content and the hemoglobin-bound content. The dissolved oxygen content is proportional to the blood Po_2. The hemoglobin-bound content depends on the total number of hemoglobin binding sites (the hemoglobin concentration) and the percent of those sites occupied by oxygen molecules (saturation). At a blood Po_2 of 150 torr, further increases in Po_2 augment only the dissolved oxygen component, since the hemoglobin binding sites are virtually fully occupied (100% saturation).

Note that for a given oxygen tension and percent saturation, the oxygen content of blood depends on the concentration of hemoglobin present. By analogy to traffic flow, the hemoglobin concentration in blood represents the number of buses carrying passengers on a highway, and the hemoglobin saturation represents the fraction of the seats on the buses that are occupied. Blood with a low hemoglobin concentration will necessarily have a low oxygen content even if the hemoglobin is fully saturated because the number of oxygen binding sites is directly related to concentration of hemoglobin. By contrast, blood with a high hemoglobin concentration and a low P_{O_2} could conceivably have a higher oxygen content than fully saturated blood in which there is a lesser hemoglobin concentration.

Carbon Monoxide

Carbon monoxide is a lipophilic molecule that combines with hemoglobin at the same heme sites where oxygen binds, forming *carboxyhemoglobin.* Figure 5–7 shows a comparison of the oxyhemoglobin and carboxyhemoglobin dissociation curves as a function of the oxygen or carbon monoxide tension in blood. Note that the affinity of hemoglobin for carbon monoxide is approximately 200 times

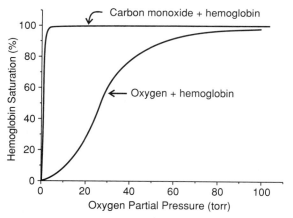

Figure 5–7. Oxyhemoglobin and carboxyhemoglobin dissociation curves. Carbon monoxide competes with oxygen for the same binding sites on hemoglobin, but with more than 200 times the affinity of oxygen. Above a blood P_{CO} of about 0.5 torr, virtually all of the hemoglobin binding sites are occupied by carbon monoxide. Note that the carboxyhemoglobin dissociation curve is hyperbolic, while the oxyhemoglobin dissociation curve is sigmoidal.

higher than that for oxygen. Consequently, if the partial pressure of carbon monoxide in blood rises above 0.5 torr, virtually all of the binding sites on hemoglobin will become occupied by carbon monoxide. This renders the hemoglobin ineffective for the transport of oxygen.

When only some of the hemoglobin binding sites are occupied by carbon monoxide, the remaining sites can still function as oxygen carriers. Figure 5–8 shows the relationship between oxygen tension and blood oxygen content for a sample of normal blood with a hemoglobin concentration of 14 g/dl and of blood with a reduced hemoglobin concentration of 7 g/dl caused by a low hematocrit (anemia). Normal and anemic blood have the same percent saturation at any given P_{O_2}, but the oxygen content is lower in anemia because the total number of hemoglobin binding sites is less. A third curve in Figure 5–8 shows the relationship between P_{O_2} and oxygen content in a blood sample with a hemoglobin concentration of 14 g/dl where 50% of the binding sites are occupied by carbon monoxide. In this situation, oxygen can occupy a maximum of 50% of the binding sites, so the physiological oxygen binding capacity is functionally reduced. In this example, note that even if the blood P_{O_2} is 100 torr, both oxyhemoglobin saturation and oxygen content will be reduced.

When carbon monoxide binds to some of the sites on hemoglobin, the relationship between P_{O_2} and oxygen saturation for the remaining sites loses its normal sigmoidal shape and becomes hyperbolic (see Figure 5–8). This change in shape interferes with oxygen unloading in the tissues because it forces the tissues to maintain a lower P_{O_2} outside the capillary to achieve the same change in oxygen content along the capillary. The lower tissue P_{O_2} then reduces the driving gradient for oxygen diffusion away from the capillary (see Chapter 6). Thus, carbon monoxide functionally reduces the ability of hemoglobin to carry oxygen and also interferes with its normal release along the capillaries.

In a healthy subject living in an urban environment, carboxyhemoglobin typically occupies 1% to 2% of the hemoglobin binding capacity. By contrast, heavy smokers may exhibit carboxyhemoglobin levels in excess of 10%. If a subject with carboxyhemoglobin is given carbon monoxide–free air to breathe, about half of the carbon monoxide will have been eliminated after 4 hours. In acciden-

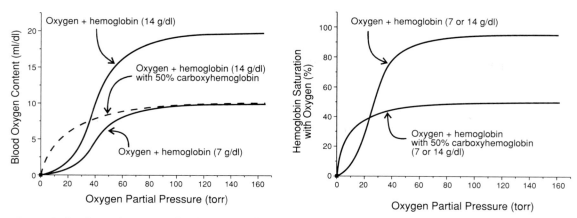

Figure 5 – 8. Effects of anemia and carbon monoxide on blood oxygen content *(left)* and hemoglobin saturation *(right)*. Blood oxygen content depends on the Po_2, the percent hemoglobin saturation, and the concentration of hemoglobin present. For example, at a concentration of 14 g/dl, hemoglobin can bind a maximum of 19.46 ml of oxygen per deciliter when fully saturated. When the concentration of hemoglobin is reduced to 7 g/dl because of a low hematocrit, the maximum oxyhemoglobin binding is reduced to 9.73 at 100% saturation. At a hemoglobin concentration of 14 g/dl, if carbon monoxide binds to 50% of the hemoglobin binding sites, the maximal oxyhemoglobin saturation is reduced to 50% and the maximal oxyhemoglobin binding is reduced to 9.73 ml/dl. Moreover, the oxyhemoglobin dissociation curve becomes hyperbolic when carbon monoxide binds to some of the sites, thereby hindering oxygen release in the systemic capillaries.

tal carbon monoxide poisoning, patients are given high concentrations of oxygen to breathe. The higher concentration of oxygen competes more effectively for hemoglobin binding sites and speeds up the rate of carbon monoxide elimination from the body. Even more rapid elimination of carbon monoxide can be achieved using a *hyperbaric chamber* to increase the barometric pressure above atmospheric. Under hyperbaric conditions arterial oxygen tensions in excess of 1,000 torr can be achieved, which hastens displacement of carbon monoxide molecules from hemoglobin binding sites and promotes their elimination.

Hemoglobin Affinity for Oxygen

The binding affinity of hemoglobin for oxygen is expressed by the *hemoglobin P_{50}*, defined as the Po_2 corresponding to a 50% oxyhemoglobin saturation. A *higher* P_{50} implies a *lower* affinity, because a higher Po_2 is needed to achieve a given oxygen saturation. Under normal conditions, adult hemoglobin is half-saturated at a Po_2 of about 27 torr. Fetal hemoglobin exhibits higher affinity for oxygen (P_{50} = 20 to 22 torr), a feature that may enhance

fetal uptake of oxygen from maternal blood (Chapter 10).

The affinity of hemoglobin for oxygen varies under physiological conditions including blood temperature, Pco_2, and pH (Figure 5 – 9). For example, decreases in blood pH below 7.4 tend to decrease the affinity of hemoglobin for oxygen (rightward shift in the oxyhemoglobin dissociation curve), while increases in pH shift the relationship to the left (increased affinity). Increases in blood temperature above 37 °C shift the dissociation curve to the right, while decreases in temperature shift the curve leftward. Finally, blood carbon dioxide tensions greater than 40 torr tend to shift the dissociation curve to the right, while reductions in Pco_2 shift the curve to the left. The effect of carbon dioxide on the affinity of hemoglobin for oxygen has been attributed to the Danish physiologist Christian Bohr and has come to be known as the *Bohr effect*.[1] Part of the Bohr effect is due to the decrease in pH that occurs as Pco_2 is increased, and part of it is caused by direct effects of carbon dioxide on the hemoglobin molecule.

[1] Interestingly, it appears that August Krogh was actually the first to note the existence of this effect.

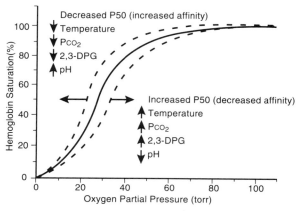

Figure 5–9. Oxyhemoglobin affinity. The affinity of hemoglobin for oxygen is expressed as the P_{50}. Increases in P_{CO_2}, temperature, or 2,3-diphosphoglycerate (2,3-DPG) or decreases in pH shift the oxyhemoglobin dissociation curve to the right (increased P_{50} = decreased affinity), while opposite changes shift the curve to the left (decreased P_{50} = increased affinity) relative to the standard value of 27 torr.

The changes in hemoglobin affinity that occur with altered temperature, carbon dioxide, and pH occur rapidly and can enhance oxygen uptake in the lung and release in the systemic tissues. For example, during exercise a working muscle produces carbon dioxide and heat and may produce lactic acid. As blood flows through muscle capillaries, oxygen diffuses out. Simultaneously, heat, carbon dioxide, and lactic acid diffuse into the blood. These factors all tend to shift the dissociation curve dynamically to the right, thereby promoting a greater amount of oxygen release from hemoglobin for a given capillary P_{O_2}. The importance of the shift in the oxyhemoglobin dissociation curve is that it augments the capillary P_{O_2}, enhancing oxygen diffusion out of the blood for a given decrease in oxygen content from arterial to venous blood. When this blood travels to the lungs and enters the pulmonary capillaries the P_{CO_2} decreases, the pH increases, and the blood temperature decreases slightly. These factors enhance the quantity of oxygen taken up into blood for a given alveolar P_{O_2}. Note that in both of the above examples, changes in hemoglobin affinity occur rapidly within the time span of a red blood cell traversing a capillary.

Red Blood Cell 2,3-Diphosphoglycerate

Mature human red blood cells synthesize the compound 2,3-diphosphoglycerate (2,3-DPG) from the glycolytic intermediate 1,3-diphosphoglycerate using the enzyme 2,3-diphosphoglycerate mutase. The 2,3-DPG remains inside the red blood cell and reduces the affinity of hemoglobin for oxygen, thus shifting the dissociation curve to the right by an amount proportional to the concentration of 2,3-DPG (see Figure 5–9). This effect on hemoglobin affinity for oxygen occurs for two reasons. First, 2,3-DPG binds directly to the hemoglobin molecule, causing a conformational change that decreases its affinity for oxygen. Second, increases in 2,3-DPG tend to lower red blood cell pH, which further promotes a rightward shift in the dissociation curve. Although the regulation of red blood cell 2,3-DPG concentration is influenced by many factors, the most important appears to be the average level of blood oxyhemoglobin saturation. Factors that reduce average blood saturation, such as chronic hypoxemia (due to lung disease or residence at high altitude), tend to augment the red blood cell 2,3-DPG concentration and cause a rightward shift in the dissociation curve. Blood bank storage of blood in acid-citrate-dextrose anticoagulant solution is associated with a gradual depletion of red blood cell 2,3-DPG concentration, causing a decrease in the P_{50} (leftward shift) of the blood over a 2-week period. The physiological importance of changes in hemoglobin P_{50} caused by changes in 2,3-DPG has been the subject of some debate. It now appears that the significance of this effect is relatively small.

CARBON DIOXIDE TRANSPORT IN BLOOD

Under resting conditions, the cells in an adult human typically produce about 200 ml of carbon dioxide per minute. To prevent its buildup in the tissues, carbon dioxide must be carried back to the lungs where it can be eliminated in exhaled gas. In this process, carbon dioxide first diffuses into capillary blood because the tissue P_{CO_2} is higher than the P_{CO_2} in arterial blood entering the capillaries. As carbon dioxide enters the capillary, the blood P_{CO_2} and carbon dioxide content increase. After traveling to the lungs, the blood passes through the pulmonary capillaries where carbon dioxide leaves the blood as it diffuses down its partial pressure gradient into alveolar gas. As this occurs, the blood P_{CO_2} and carbon dioxide content again decrease. Under resting conditions, systemic arterial blood normally has a P_{CO_2} of about 40 torr, while blood returning to the lungs has a P_{CO_2} of about 47 torr.

Carbon dioxide is carried in three different forms in blood. Most of the carbon dioxide in blood is carried in the form of *bicarbonate ions.* Bicarbonate ions are formed directly from the hydroxylation of carbon dioxide by water inside the red blood cells:

$$H^+OH^- + CO_2 \longleftrightarrow HCO_3^- + H^+ \quad (1)$$

The velocity of this reaction is accelerated about 12,000 times by the enzyme *carbonic anhydrase,* which is present within the red blood cells. Because there is virtually no carbonic anhydrase in the plasma, most of the bicarbonate in blood is formed within the red blood cells.

Carbon dioxide is also carried in chemical combination with hemoglobin, at a different site than where oxygen is bound. At the amino terminus of the α and β hemoglobin chains, carbon dioxide can reversibly combine to form a *carbamino compound* while releasing a proton:

$$R - NH_3 + CO_2 \longleftrightarrow R - COO^- + H^+ \quad (2)$$

The third mechanism available for carbon dioxide transport is in dissolved form. The dissolved carbon dioxide content is proportional to the P_{CO_2}. Although carbon dioxide is more soluble in plasma than oxygen, it is still relatively insoluble so, and relatively less carbon dioxide is carried in this form. Note, however, that all three forms of carbon dioxide carriage exist in equilibrium in a sample of blood obtained from the aorta or pulmonary artery.

Figure 5–10 shows the overall relationship between partial pressure and carbon dioxide content in a sample of arterial blood. The *total carbon dioxide content* in a blood sample reflects the sum of the dissolved carbamino and bicarbonate contributions. Although nearly all of the bicarbonate is made in the red blood cells, much of this enters the plasma in exchange for chloride ions through a coupled ion transporter in the red blood cell membrane. Consequently, more bicarbonate is carried in the

plasma than in the red blood cells. The exchange of bicarbonate and chloride ions between the red blood cell and the plasma is known as the *chloride shift.*

As oxygen is unloaded from blood along the peripheral capillaries, the dissociation curve for carbon dioxide is shifted upward (Figure 5–11), allowing the blood to take up more carbon dioxide content at any given P_{CO_2}. The shift is caused by an enhanced ability of deoxygenated hemoglobin to form carbamino compounds and an enhanced ability of deoxygenated hemoglobin to buffer hydrogen ions released during the formation of bicarbonate and carbamino compounds (see equations 1 and 2 above). Since more deoxygenated hemoglobin is formed as oxygen is released, this effect increases the amount of carbon dioxide that can be taken up by the blood at any given P_{CO_2}. It occurs rapidly enough so that the curve can shift dynamically as oxygen is unloaded along a capillary, analogous to the shift in the oxyhemoglobin dissociation curve due to the effects of changing P_{CO_2}. Thus, the unloading of oxygen from hemoglobin enhances the ability of the blood to take up carbon dioxide. This process is reversed in the lung, where the uptake of oxygen along the pulmonary capillaries shifts the

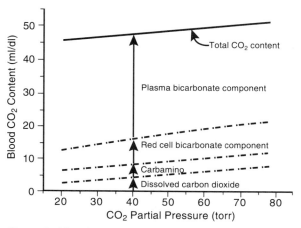

Figure 5–10. Relationship between P_{CO_2} and blood carbon dioxide concentration (the "carbon dioxide dissociation curve") in fully oxygenated blood. The total carbon dioxide content *(solid line)* reflects the sum of dissolved carbon dioxide content, carbamino content, bicarbonate inside red blood cells, and bicarbonate in the plasma *(dotted lines).*

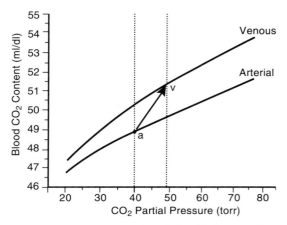

Figure 5–11. Changes in the relationship between P_{CO_2} and blood carbon dioxide content when the blood is partially deoxygenated. Arterial line shows the carbon dioxide dissociation curve in oxygenated blood (same as in Fig. 5–10); venous line shows the changes in the curve when oxyhemoglobin saturation is reduced to 75%. Deoxygenation shifts the composite carbon dioxide content curve upward, owing mostly to the enhanced carbamino uptake. Arrow shows the change in carbon dioxide content that occurs as arterial blood (P_{CO_2} = 40 torr, O_2 saturation = 98%) passes through systemic capillaries and becomes venous blood (P_{CO_2} = 47 torr, O_2 saturation = 75%). This facilitates a greater change in CO_2 content for a given increase in P_{CO_2}.

carbon dioxide dissociation curve downward, thereby unloading more carbon dioxide content for a given alveolar P_{CO_2}. The effect of changes in oxyhemoglobin saturation on the relationship of the carbon dioxide content to P_{CO_2} is referred to as the *Haldane effect,* after the 19th century physiologist J. S. Haldane.

E X A M P L E. Blood passing through the lungs of a resting subject undergoes a decrease in P_{CO_2} of 7 torr (47 → 40). This is associated with a decrease in carbon dioxide content from 54 to 49 ml/dl. If the metabolic production of carbon dioxide ($\dot{V}_{CO_2}$) is 225 ml/min, what is this subject's cardiac output?

Note that the Fick equation can be applied to carbon dioxide as well as to oxygen. From this equation

$$\dot{Q}t = \frac{\dot{V}_{CO_2}}{(C\bar{v}_{CO_2} - Ca_{CO_2})}$$

where $C\bar{v}_{CO_2}$ and Ca_{CO_2} are the carbon dioxide con-

tents of mixed venous and arterial blood (in ml/dl), and $\dot{Q}t$ is the cardiac output (in dl/min). Thus,

$$\dot{Q}t = 225/5 = 45 \text{ dl/min} = 4.5 \text{ liters/min.} \quad \blacksquare$$

INTERACTIONS OF OXYGEN AND CARBON DIOXIDE TRANSPORT

Figure 5–12 summarizes the events that take place in a red blood cell and the surrounding plasma as blood moves through a systemic capillary. Carbon dioxide in the tissue diffuses down its partial pressure gradient into the plasma. Some carbon dioxide molecules remain in the plasma as dissolved carbon dioxide, whereas others diffuse farther into the red blood cell where they meet up with one of three fates. Although a small amount may remain in dissolved form in the red blood cell, most of the carbon dioxide molecules are hydrated into bicarbonate and hydrogen ions by carbonic anhydrase. As the concentration of bicarbonate ions in the red blood cell begins to increase, bicarbonate is transported through the cell membrane in exchange for chloride ions through a coupled membrane transporter. Positively charged hydrogen ions do not cross the cell membrane readily and are instead buffered by hemoglobin (chiefly through the imidazole rings on histidine). Other carbon dioxide molecules bind to the amino terminus of hemoglobin α and β chains, forming carbamino groups. While all of this is happening, oxygen diffuses down its partial pressure gradient from the red blood cell into the plasma and from the plasma into the tissue. As oxygen diffuses out of the cells, more oxygen dissociates from hemoglobin as it attempts to remain in equilibrium with the changing P_{O_2} in plasma. Note that the hydrogen ions released by the hydration of carbon dioxide and the increase in P_{CO_2} in the red blood cell both tend to alter the shape of the hemoglobin molecule, causing its affinity for oxygen to decrease. This change shifts the oxyhemoglobin dissociation curve to the right, promoting the release of more oxygen at any given P_{O_2} (the Bohr effect). As the hemoglobin saturation decreases, two important changes take place. First, desaturated hemoglobin is more effective at buffering hydrogen ions than oxygenated hemoglobin. This promotes the production of bicarbonate in the red blood cell, because it re-

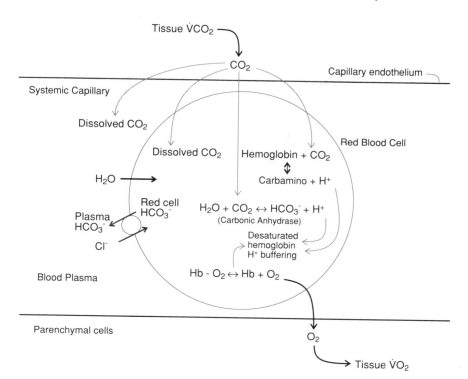

Figure 5–12. Summary of events that occur as a red blood cell passes through a systemic capillary. Oxygen unloading along the capillary is enhanced by increases in P_{CO_2} and decreases in pH (the Bohr effect), while carbon dioxide loading into blood is enhanced by the simultaneous desaturation of hemoglobin (the Haldane effect). Most of the oxygen is bound to hemoglobin in the red blood cells, whereas most of the bicarbonate produced in the red blood cells is transported to the plasma. See text for further explanation.

duces the accumulation of free hydrogen ions released by the carbon dioxide hydration reaction. Second, deoxygenated hemoglobin is better able to form carbamino compounds, so the uptake of carbon dioxide as carbamino is enhanced. [These changes mediate the Haldane effect.] Finally, water moves into the red blood cell in response to the increase in the number of osmotically active ions present and the cell swells slightly. This entire set of processes reverses direction as the blood passes through the pulmonary circulation, where oxygen is loaded into blood, and carbon dioxide is unloaded.

The above reactions occur very rapidly and are nearly complete within the short time that it takes a red blood cell to pass through a capillary. After the cell leaves the capillary, a small amount of additional equilibration of bicarbonate continues to occur between the plasma and cell, owing to the limited speed of the cell membrane bicarbonate–chloride transporter. This effect causes minor changes in postcapillary P_{CO_2} and pH. However, complete equilibration between red blood cells and plasma is again restored within 2 seconds after the blood exits the end of the capillary.

Chapter 6

Diffusion

Diffusion is a transport process by which gas moves from one region to another. Respiratory gases diffuse from regions of higher partial pressure to regions of lower partial pressure because their molecules are continuously in motion and because it is energetically favorable to do so. Thus, without a partial pressure difference there can be no net movement of gas by diffusion. Diffusion is a passive process because it occurs without the need for energy expenditure.

In the airspaces of the lungs, diffusion is the primary mechanism responsible for gas transport from the distal airways to the alveolar-capillary membrane, which separates capillary blood from alveolar gas. Diffusion is also the mechanism responsible for gas transport through the alveolar-capillary membrane that separates alveolar gas from pulmonary capillary blood. In the systemic capillaries, diffusion is the process by which oxygen moves from capillary blood to the cells, where it is consumed in the mitochondria. It is also the mechanism by which carbon dioxide produced in the cells moves out of the tissue into the blood.

Gas Diffusion in Alveoli

As inspired air moves from the central airways toward the alveoli, the total cross-sectional area of the airways increases dramatically (see Figure 2–3). Consequently, the forward velocity of inspired air decreases progressively as it moves into the lungs. By the time the air reaches the terminal airspaces in the lung, diffusion becomes the primary mechanism for transporting gas to the alveolar epithelial surface. Diffusion of gases between alveoli can also occur through small pores in the interalveolar septa. Called *pores of Kohn*, these interalveolar pathways may help to reduce differences in alveolar gas tensions between adjacent lung regions. By allowing diffusion of gases between alveoli, the pores of Kohn also permit some ventilation to reach alveoli whose airways may be blocked by mucus or other material.

Diffusion of Gases Dissolved in Liquids

Diffusion occurs from regions of higher partial pressure to lower partial pressure. Consider the situation in which a layer of liquid (effectively a membrane) separates two regions containing different partial pressures of a gas (Figure 6–1). Fick's law summarizes the factors that influence the rate of diffusion of the gas through the liquid barrier:

$$\dot{V} = \frac{Ad}{T}(P_1 - P_2) \qquad (1)$$

where $\dot{V}$ is the volume of gas diffusing across the membrane per unit time (ml/min), A is the surface area available for diffusion (cm^2), T is the thickness of the membrane (cm), and $(P_1 - P_2)$ is the gas partial pressure difference across the membrane (torr). In this equation, d (cm^2/torr/min) is called the *diffusion coefficient* and is related to the solubility of the gas within the membrane and the square root of the molecular weight of the gas.

Other factors held constant, doubling the partial pressure difference between the two regions will double the flow (i.e., the volume of gas crossing the membrane per unit time). Thus, the rate of gas transport by diffusion (ml/min) is proportional to the partial pressure difference (ΔP, in torr). It is also proportional to the surface area available for diffusion since doubling the surface area will double the volume of gas crossing the barrier per unit time

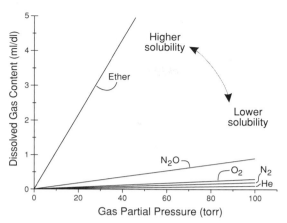

Figure 6–2. Relationship between the volume of gas dissolved in a liquid and the partial pressure of the gas in the liquid. The slope of the line is the solubility of the gas in the liquid. Gases that do not combine chemically with the liquid exhibit linear relationships (constant solubility at a given temperature).

(other factors held constant). The diffusive gas transport is inversely proportional to the thickness of the membrane; doubling the thickness will halve the flow rate across the membrane. The last term (d) influencing the rate of diffusion is a function of the solubility of the gas in the barrier and the molecular weight of the gas.

The *solubility* is defined as the volume of gas (ml) that must be dissolved in 100 ml of the barrier liquid to raise the partial pressure in it by 1 torr. Figure 6–2 is a plot of the content of gas dissolved in a saline solution (milliliters of dissolved gas per deciliter of liquid) at different partial pressures of the gas. When the solubility of a gas in the membrane is large, gas will diffuse at a faster rate through the membrane. One way to think of this is to imagine the events at the surface of the membrane, where gas molecules are diffusing from one side to the other. To get through the membrane, gas molecules first must impact on the surface and become dissolved in the barrier material. The molecules then diffuse through and exit from the far side (see Fig. 6–1). If the gas is highly soluble in the barrier, it will become dissolved in the barrier more readily than an insoluble gas. The dependence of diffusion on molecular weight relates to the velocity of the molecular motion in a gas. At a given temperature, gas molecules have the same average kinetic energy (½

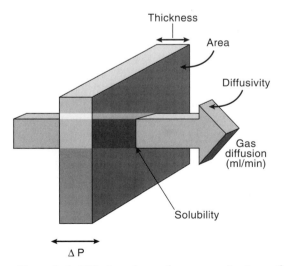

Figure 6–1. Diffusion of a gas from one region to another through a barrier. Fick's law of diffusion describes the factors influencing the rate of gas diffusion from a region of high partial pressure to a region with lower partial pressure.

mv^2, where m is mass and v is velocity). Thus, two gas molecules with the same kinetic energy will have velocities that are inversely proportional to the square roots of their molecular weights. Hence, heavier molecular weight gases diffuse more slowly than lighter gases as a consequence of their slower molecular velocities.

EQUILIBRATION BETWEEN ALVEOLAR GAS AND CAPILLARY BLOOD

The lung contains approximately 300 million alveoli, each of which is roughly spherical and has a diameter of about 1/3 mm. Thus, the surface area available for gas exchange between alveolar gas and pulmonary capillary blood is about 100 m^2. Blood normally enters the pulmonary capillaries with a mixed venous oxygen tension ($P\bar{v}_{O_2}$) of approximately 40 torr and a P_{CO_2} of about 47 torr. As the blood enters the capillaries, oxygen and carbon dioxide diffuse across the alveolar blood–gas barrier because the partial pressures in mixed venous blood and alveolar gas are different. Because the P_{CO_2} in alveolar gas (PA_{CO_2}) is normally maintained at about 40 torr by the flow of fresh gas in (alveolar ventilation) and the alveolar P_{O_2} is normally around 100 torr, the equilibration along the capillary causes the P_{CO_2} to decrease and the P_{O_2} to increase in capillary blood. Normally, blood exiting from the end of the pulmonary capillary has the same P_{O_2} and P_{CO_2} as alveolar gas. The following sections examine the process of gas exchange along the capillary, beginning with the simplest case of inert gas transfer.

Physiologically Inert Gases

In understanding the events driving diffusion of gases between pulmonary capillary blood and alveolar gas, consider first the case of a gas such as helium, which does not combine chemically with blood and has a linear content–partial pressure relationship (Figure 6–2). This gas is relatively insoluble in blood. Figure 6–3A shows the sequence of events that might occur in a single alveolus after a subject inhales a single breath of helium, which suddenly increases the alveolar helium partial pressure (P_{He}) to 300 torr. At that instant, blood entering the pulmonary capillary contains no dissolved helium, and the partial pressure difference between alveolar gas and blood at the beginning of the capillary is 300 torr (300 − 0 torr). Driven by this ΔP, helium diffuses into the blood, and the partial pressure in a small volume element of blood at the capillary entrance begins to increase. As that element moves through the capillary, the ΔP between it and alveolar gas decreases because its partial pressure increases. [Note that the volume of alveolar gas decreases slightly but the alveolar helium tension remains at 300 torr.] A short distance into the capillary, the helium partial pressure in this element has increased to 300 torr. At this point the ΔP is zero, and no more helium is exchanged for this element along the remainder of the capillary. [Obviously, helium is still being taken up at the beginning of the capillary as new blood elements enter.] Although this element will remain in the capillary for about 0.75 second, virtually all of the gas exchange is completed in the early part of the capillary. Hence, the remainder of the time spent there does not contribute further to gas exchange. Gas exchange is said to be *perfusion limited* in this example, because blood leaving the capillary has reached equilibrium with alveolar gas.

Consider another example in which the subject has just inhaled a trace amount of the anesthetic gas ether, causing the alveolar partial pressure of ether to increase to 0.001 torr (see Figure 6–3B). Ether has a relatively high solubility in blood (see Figure 6–2). Once again, blood entering the pulmonary capillary contains no ether, so an element of blood encounters a ΔP of 0.001 torr as it enters the capillary. This causes ether to diffuse into the element of blood, causing its partial pressure to rise. As before, the partial pressure of ether in this element increases to 0.001 torr soon after it enters the capillary, and no subsequent exchange of ether occurs for this element. This uptake is also perfusion limited.

In both examples, the *rate of equilibration* between alveolar gas and the blood element was sufficiently rapid to permit essentially complete equilibration in less than the 0.75 second it spent in the capillary. Note that the volume of gas (in milliliters) entering the blood may have differed in the two examples, as did the magnitude of the changes in blood partial pressure. However, the time required to reach equilibrium was less than the time spent in the capillary. The rapid rate of equilibration for

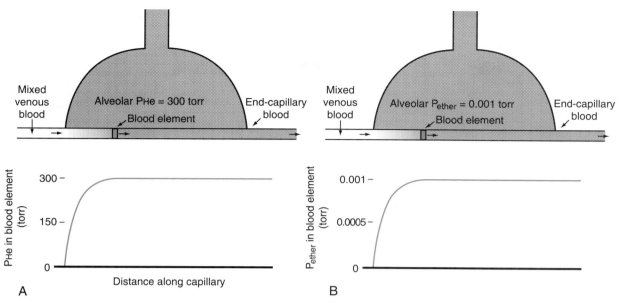

Figure 6-3. Inert gas transfer between alveolar gas and pulmonary capillary blood. *A.* The change in partial pressure of helium (PHe) within a small element of blood as it passes along a pulmonary capillary. Alveolar PHe remains constant at 300 torr, and blood entering the capillary contains no dissolved helium. Equilibration between alveolar gas and this element occurs very rapidly, and equilibrium is reached soon after the element enters the capillary. *B.* The change in partial pressure of the anesthetic gas ether in a small element of blood as it passes along a pulmonary capillary. Alveolar ether tension remains constant at 0.001 torr, and blood entering the capillary contains no dissolved ether. Equilibration between alveolar gas and blood is also achieved long before the element reaches the end of the capillary. Gas uptake is perfusion limited in both cases.

these gases is a consequence of their solubility in the blood–gas barrier, relative to their solubility in blood. In both of the examples the gas solubility in the blood–gas barrier was similar to the solubility in blood, so the ratio of these terms was close to unity. Much slower rates of equilibration would have occurred if the solubility of the gas in blood was much higher than in the membrane, as is the case for carbon monoxide, and, to a lesser extent, oxygen and carbon dioxide.

Carbon Monoxide, Oxygen, and Carbon Dioxide Equilibration Along the Pulmonary Capillary

Oxygen, carbon dioxide, and carbon monoxide all combine chemically with blood, giving rise to the nonlinear partial pressure versus content relationships seen for these gases. Note that the slope of this relationship for any gas is its *effective solubility*. For example, the effective solubility of oxygen in blood

is low at partial pressures greater than about 100 torr but increases markedly at P_{O_2} values less than about 60 torr because the curve becomes steeper (Figure 6–4). The solubility of carbon dioxide in blood is much higher than that of oxygen because its slope is steeper, but its solubility varies less as the partial pressure varies (i.e., the relationship is more linear). Because the slope of the partial pressure–content relationship for carbon monoxide is very steep at tensions below 1 to 2 torr, the effective solubility of carbon monoxide is enormous in blood in this range.

Consider the events that would occur along an alveolar capillary if a subject inhaled a breath containing trace amounts of carbon monoxide and increased the alveolar partial pressure of carbon monoxide to 0.1 torr. Assuming that mixed venous blood contains no carbon monoxide, blood entering the pulmonary capillary would encounter a ΔP of 0.1 torr, and carbon monoxide would diffuse into the

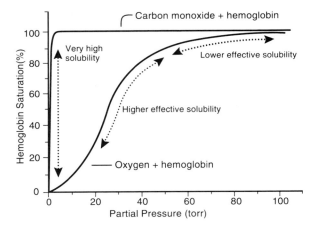

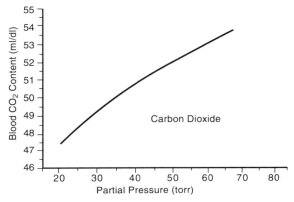

Figure 6–4. Contents of oxygen, carbon monoxide, and carbon dioxide as a function of their partial pressure in blood. The effective solubility of each gas in blood is equivalent to the slope of the line at any point. Thus, oxygen is highly soluble at partial pressures of 20 to 60 torr but relatively insoluble above 100 torr (where most of the hemoglobin binding sites are occupied). Carbon dioxide is much more soluble in blood than is oxygen (steeper slope). Unlike oxygen, its solubility is relatively constant as a function of partial pressure. At a partial pressure of less than 1 torr, effective carbon monoxide solubility is extremely large. At partial pressures greater than 1 torr, carbon monoxide content increases by adding dissolved carbon monoxide only, and its solubility is small.

blood. However, as shown in Figure 6–5A, the partial pressure in an element of blood would rise slowly as it moved through the capillary and still would not have reached the alveolar level by the end of the capillary. In this example, alveolar carbon monoxide was still exchanging with blood at

the end of the capillary and would have continued if the element had spent more time in the capillary. Hence, gas exchange in this situation is said to be *diffusion limited.*

Why is gas exchange perfusion limited in some cases and diffusion limited in others? The answer arises from the fact that the gases entering (or leaving) blood must diffuse through the blood–gas barrier. Gases that do not combine chemically with blood (e.g., helium, argon, nitrogen, anesthetic gases, and other physiologically inert gases) exhibit a similar solubility in the blood gas membranes and in blood. When the ratio of these solubilities is close to unity, the gas exhibits a rapid rate of equilibration along the capillary. By contrast, gases that combine chemically with blood (e.g., oxygen, carbon dioxide, and carbon monoxide) have a much higher effective solubility in blood than in the membrane. Consequently, their rate of equilibration along the capillary is slower. In the case of carbon monoxide, the low solubility in the membrane combined with an enormous solubility in blood causes such a slow rate of equilibration that carbon monoxide exchange is always diffusion limited. Note that carbon monoxide uptake in an isolated lung perfused with plasma (no red blood cells) would be perfusion limited, since carbon monoxide has a similar low solubility in plasma and the blood–gas barrier.

The rate of equilibration between alveolar gas and capillary blood is analogous to loading railroad hopper cars with coal through a chute (Figure 6–6). If the train cars move along at a speed such that each car spends 0.75 second under the chute, the cars will be completely filled in the time allotted (perfusion limited uptake) (Figure 6–6A) if the size of the chute (analogous to the solubility of the gas in the membrane) is well matched to the size of each car (the solubility in blood). In this situation, additional time spent under the chute will not result in additional loading, since the cars will already be completely filled. By contrast, if the chute is small (low membrane solubility) and each car is large (high blood solubility), then the cars will leave before they have filled completely (Figure 6–6B) (diffusion limitation).

How do oxygen and carbon dioxide fit into this picture? These physiological gases have high effective solubilities in blood owing to their chemical combination but relatively low solubilities in the

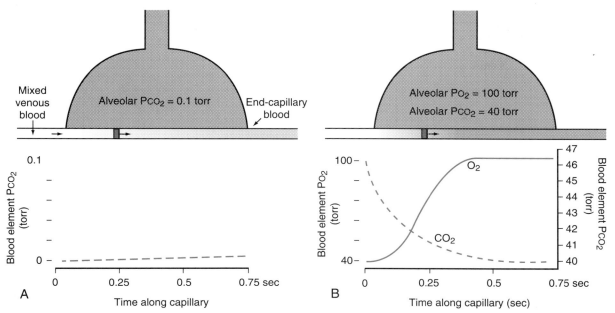

Figure 6–5. Physiological gas transfer between alveolar gas and pulmonary capillary blood. *A.* Partial pressure of carbon monoxide in an element of blood passing through a pulmonary capillary. Alveolar Pco remains constant at 0.1 torr, and mixed venous blood enters without any carboxyhemoglobin. Exchange of carbon monoxide is still occurring as the element leaves the end of the capillary because its rate of equilibration is slow relative to the time spent in the capillary. *B.* Oxygen and carbon dioxide partial pressures in an element of blood passing through a pulmonary capillary. Mixed venous blood enters the capillary with $Po_2 = 40$ and $Pco_2 = 47$ torr. Gas diffusion proceeds rapidly enough so that equilibration with alveolar gas is achieved before the end of the capillary.

blood–gas barrier. Hence, both of these gases equilibrate more slowly than physiologically inert gases. However, their rate of equilibration is still rapid enough to allow complete equilibration before the end of the capillary. Figure 6–5*B* shows the time course of changes in oxygen and carbon dioxide in an element of blood passing through the pulmonary capillary. Normally, equilibration of these gases is complete in about 0.25 second—about a third of the way along the capillary. According to Fick's law of diffusion, carbon dioxide should diffuse through water about 20 times faster than oxygen, based on its greater solubility in water. However, both oxygen and carbon dioxide equilibrate at about the same rate because the larger diffusion coefficient for carbon dioxide is counterbalanced by its lower membrane–blood solubility ratio. This is why oxygen and carbon dioxide take about the same amount of time to reach equilibration along the pulmonary capillaries.

Does Diffusion Ever Limit Oxygen or Carbon Dioxide Exchange?

Exercise. Normally, the exchange of oxygen and carbon dioxide in the lung is perfusion limited. During strenuous exercise, the time that an element of blood spends in a pulmonary capillary decreases because capillary blood velocity increases. Since the rate of equilibration between alveolar gas and capillary blood does not increase, equilibration between gas and blood is not reached until farther along the capillary. In some healthy conditioned athletes, the increase in cardiac output at high levels of exercise can shorten the capillary transit time to less than about 0.25 second (Figure 6–7). If this happens, blood leaves the pulmonary capillaries before oxygen and carbon dioxide have fully equilibrated with alveolar gas. When this occurs, the exchange of these gases becomes diffusion limited. As a result, blood leaves the lungs with a Po_2 that is a few torr

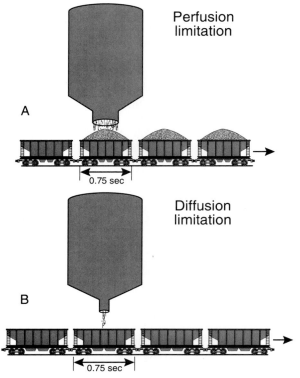

Figure 6–6. Gas transfer across the blood–gas barrier. The rate at which alveolar gas and blood equilibrate depends on the solubility of the gas in the blood–gas barrier (diameter of the coal chute) relative to the effective solubility in blood (size of the railroad cars). Each car spends 0.75 second under the chute before moving on. *A.* Membrane solubility is well matched to the solubility in blood, so the cars leaving the dock are filled fully (perfusion limitation). *B.* Membrane solubility is low while blood solubility is high, and the cars leave without being completely filled (diffusion limitation).

lower than alveolar gas and a Pco_2 that is slightly higher than alveolar gas. This effect is measurable but occurs only at extremely high levels of exercise.

High Altitude. At high altitude, ambient air still contains 20.9% oxygen but the barometric pressure decreases. Thus, the inspired Po_2 and alveolar Po_2 will decrease, producing arterial hypoxemia (low arterial Po_2) even if the lungs are healthy. When arterial blood hemoglobin is desaturated because the alveolar Po_2 is low, the effective solubility of oxygen in blood is increased. (Note that a line connecting the arterial and mixed venous points on the oxyhemoglobin dissociation curve is steeper than when arterial blood is fully saturated.) Since the

solubility of oxygen in the blood–gas barrier does not change, this slows the rate of equilibration for oxygen along the capillaries. In healthy subjects who exercise (thereby shortening capillary transit time) at high altitudes, this can cause oxygen exchange to become diffusion limited. Again, the diffusion limitation is caused by the slow rate of equilibration—not the lower alveolar Po_2 itself.

Lung Diseases. Pathological changes in diseased lungs can have profound effects on the efficiency with which those lungs exchange gases. Thickening of the alveolar capillary membrane, as occurs in interstitial fibrosis, theoretically could impair gas diffusion in the lungs and cause oxygen and carbon dioxide exchange to become limited by diffusion. In practice, this amounts to only a small part of the lung gas exchange disturbance seen in these patients. Ventilation–perfusion inequality (see Chap-

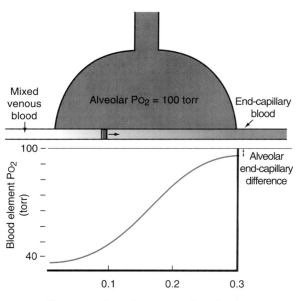

Figure 6–7. Partial pressure of oxygen in an element of blood passing through a pulmonary capillary during strenuous exercise in a highly trained athlete. Alveolar tension of oxygen remains constant at about 100 torr, and mixed venous blood enters with a Po_2 of less than 30 torr. Exchange proceeds at a normal rate, but the time spent in the capillary is less than 0.75 second, because cardiac output is very high. Hence, blood may leave the end of the capillary without quite reaching equilibrium with alveolar gas. In this situation, oxygen exchange has become diffusion limited.

ter 7) is the principal cause of the low arterial P_{O_2} often found in these patients.

In diseases such as emphysema, marked decrease in the surface area available for diffusion occurs as a result of the destruction of alveolar septal walls. This contributes to a marked reduction in the measurement of carbon monoxide diffusing capacity (see later). However, oxygen and carbon dioxide exchange remains perfusion limited in these patients.

GAS DIFFUSION IN SYSTEMIC CAPILLARIES

The unloading and loading of oxygen and carbon dioxide in the systemic capillaries also occurs by passive diffusion. Unlike the situation in the lung, oxygen and carbon dioxide exchange in systemic capillaries may be thought of as diffusion limited under normal conditions; a greater amount of oxygen would be extracted from an element of blood if it spent more time in the capillary and more carbon dioxide would be loaded on. Systemic tissues can be modeled as a collection of individual capillaries, each of which is responsible for supplying the cylinder of cells that surround them (Figure 6–8). Outside the central capillary, consumption of oxygen by the cells causes the local P_{O_2} to decrease steeply as a

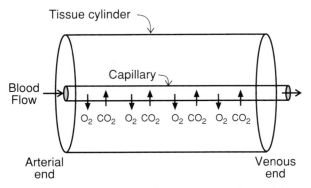

Figure 6–8. The systemic capillary–tissue cylinder model. Systemic tissues can be thought of as collections of capillaries, each of which supplies the cylinder of tissue surrounding it. The oxygen tension decreases along the capillary as oxygen diffuses into the tissue. Because it is consumed in the tissue, the oxygen tension decreases as a function of distance away from the capillary. Thus, the cells farthest from the capillary at the venous end of the cylinder are the first to encounter anoxia if the oxygen delivery into the cylinder is abnormally reduced.

function of the distance away from the capillary. If the intercapillary distances are sufficiently large, or if the blood P_{O_2} is sufficiently small, the tissue P_{O_2} may decrease to zero (*anoxia*) at sites far from the capillaries, because all of the oxygen leaving the blood is consumed before it diffuses into those regions. Note that the first cells to encounter this problem would be those farthest away from the capillary at its venous end (where the partial pressure driving diffusion out of the capillary is lowest). However, under normal conditions, the rate of diffusion within the tissue is rapid enough, and the venous P_{O_2} is great enough to ensure that the amount of oxygen reaching all cells is adequate to meet their metabolic needs. Many tissues respond to a lower arterial P_{O_2} by recruiting additional capillaries, since only a fraction of the capillaries may be receiving blood flow normally. For example, skeletal muscle may perfuse less than 20% of the capillaries at rest, but virtually all of the capillaries during exercise. This way, the intercapillary distance is decreased, allowing the tissues to extract more oxygen before diffusion begins to limit oxygen delivery to some tissue regions.

The oxygen consumption rate of tissues normally is determined by metabolic activity. If the oxygen delivery (product of blood flow and arterial oxygen content) to a tissue is reduced by lowering its blood flow, a greater percentage of the oxygen will be extracted from blood. Thus, the venous P_{O_2} and oxygen content will decrease. In this manner, tissues are able to maintain a fixed level of oxygen consumption despite physiological variability in the level of cardiac output or arterial oxygen content. This relationship can be expressed by the Fick equation of mass balance, which states that the oxygen consumption ($\dot{V}_{O_2}$, ml/min) is equal to the difference between the oxygen delivery (product of blood flow and arterial oxygen content) and the oxygen returning from tissue in venous blood (product of blood flow and venous oxygen content) (see Chapter 5).

If the systemic oxygen delivery is reduced below a critical minimum level, oxygen consumption will begin to decrease as regions of tissue anoxia develop. For whole body, this critical point generally occurs at an oxygen delivery of about 8 ml/min/kg of body weight. Figure 6–9 shows this relationship schematically. Over a wide range of oxygen deliveries, tissue oxygen uptake is relatively constant and

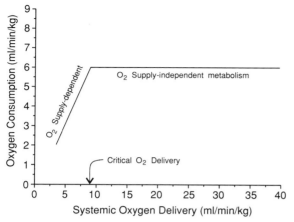

Figure 6–9. The relationship between oxygen delivery and oxygen consumption in whole-body or isolated tissues. Oxygen consumption by tissues is set by metabolic activity as long as systemic oxygen transport exceeds a critical minimum level. In the supply-independent range, changes in oxygen delivery (cardiac output · arterial oxygen content) do not alter oxygen uptake ($\dot{V}o_2$) because the fraction of oxygen extracted from blood changes reciprocally. Below a critical delivery threshold, further reductions in oxygen delivery are associated with a fall in $\dot{V}o_2$ because regions of tissue anoxia develop.

independent of oxygen supplied to the tissue. Below the critical delivery threshold, oxygen consumption decreases with further reductions in oxygen delivery (supply-dependent oxygen consumption) because regions that are anoxic cannot consume oxygen. When this occurs, lactic acid is produced by anoxic cells that must rely on anaerobic glycolysis for their entire energetic needs.

CLINICAL MEASUREMENT OF LUNG DIFFUSING CAPACITY

Theory

Recall from Fick's law of diffusion that the rate of gas diffusion through a membrane is proportional to the partial pressure difference:

$$\dot{V} = \frac{Ad}{T} \Delta P \qquad (1)$$

For the lung, the term Ad/T represents an effective *conductance* (1/resistance) for gas transfer from al-

veolus to blood, where A is the area available for diffusion in the entire lung, T is the average thickness of the barrier, and d is a function of the specific gas. When applied to the whole lung, this conductance term (Ad/T) is called the *diffusing capacity* (DL). One could measure the diffusing capacity of a gas to assess the diffusion properties of the lung if the rate of gas uptake ($\dot{V}$) is measured and the ΔP across the membrane is known. In practice, the average ΔP is difficult to determine for gases such as oxygen because the average capillary Po_2 cannot be measured (Figure 6–5B). However, the characteristics of carbon monoxide provide a solution to this problem. Because the rate of carbon monoxide equilibration along the capillary is very slow, the capillary blood partial pressure of carbon monoxide remains close to zero as small amounts of carbon monoxide are taken up (Figure 6–5A). Therefore, the ΔP for carbon monoxide can be determined by measuring the average partial pressure of carbon monoxide in alveolar gas. From Fick's law of diffusion:

$$\dot{V}_{CO} \text{ (ml/min)} = \Delta P \frac{Ad}{T} \qquad (2)$$

Thus

$$\dot{V}_{CO} = D_{L_{CO}}(P_{ACO} - P_{BLOOD_{CO}}) \qquad (3)$$

where $D_{L_{CO}}$ is the diffusing capacity $= \dfrac{Ad}{T}$, P_{ACO} is the average alveolar carbon monoxide partial pressure, and $P_{BLOOD_{CO}}$ is the average capillary blood carbon monoxide partial pressure. Since the average blood carbon monoxide tension is assumed to be zero,

$$D_{L_{CO}} = \frac{\dot{V}_{CO}}{P_{ACO}}. \qquad (4)$$

This equation says that the conductance (1/resistance) of carbon monoxide into blood is equal to the rate (ml/min) at which carbon monoxide is taken up divided by the average partial pressure difference (torr) (Figure 6–10).

Part of the "resistance" to gas uptake is caused by the alveolar-capillary membrane, and the remainder is composed of the resistance to diffusion

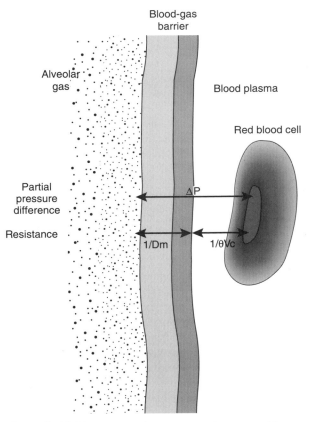

Figure 6–10. The amount of oxygen or carbon monoxide taken up by the lungs per unit time (ml/min) depends on the average partial pressure between alveolar gas and the red blood cell (ΔP) and the total resistance to gas uptake. The total resistance to gas uptake consists of a membrane resistance ($1/D_M$) plus a resistance to uptake into the red blood cell ($1/(\theta V_C)$). Factors that increase membrane thickness or reduce the capillary blood volume or hemoglobin concentration therefore will decrease the diffusing capacity for carbon monoxide.

into the red blood cell and its finite rate of combination with hemoglobin. Thus, the total resistance is the sum of these two components:

$$\frac{1}{D_{L_{CO}}} = \frac{1}{D_M} + \frac{1}{\theta V_C} \qquad (5)$$

where $1/D_{L_{CO}}$ is the total resistance to gas uptake, $1/D_M$ is the membrane resistance, and $1/\theta V_C$ is the resistance encountered in diffusing through the plasma into the red blood cell and combining with hemoglobin. These two resistances are *additive* be-

cause gas entering or leaving blood encounters them sequentially (i.e., in series). Both terms contribute about equally to the total resistance to gas uptake. The $1/\theta V_C$ term is a function of the volume of blood in the capillaries (V_C, ml) and the rate at which the gas can combine with hemoglobin (θ, in ml/(min · torr · ml blood)). The term θ is based on experimental measurements and varies with the saturation of hemoglobin (θ is greater when oxyhemoglobin saturation is less) and the hemoglobin concentration in blood (θ is greater when the hematocrit is greater). Thus, the diffusing capacity measurement is also influenced by factors other than the thickness of the membrane.

Application

To measure the diffusing capacity for carbon monoxide, a patient inhales a known concentration of carbon monoxide (typically 0.3%) plus helium (typically 10%) from residual volume to total lung capacity (TLC). After holding a breath for 10 seconds at TLC the patient exhales. The initial 500 to 1000 ml of exhaled gas contains dead space gas and is discarded. A representative sample of alveolar gas is obtained from late in the exhalation, and the P_{He} and P_{CO} are measured. Little helium is absorbed while the breath is being held because it is relatively insoluble in blood, and the exhaled helium concentration can be used to calculate the initial alveolar P_{CO} and the lung volume (the inhaled volume of helium is known; see Chapter 1). From the length of time that the breath was held and the difference between inhaled and exhaled amounts of carbon monoxide, the volume of carbon monoxide taken up can be calculated. This is divided by the average P_{CO} in alveolar gas, yielding the diffusing capacity in units of $\dfrac{ml/min}{torr}$.

Because the value of θ varies with the hemoglobin concentration, the $D_{L_{CO}}$ measurement will be less than the predicted normal value in an individual with anemia (low hematocrit). Hence, $D_{L_{CO}}$ values are usually corrected for the hemoglobin concentration. Exercise or changes in body position also can influence the $D_{L_{CO}}$ by changing the number of pulmonary capillaries receiving blood flow, thereby changing both the surface area and the capillary blood volume (V_C). Breathing supplemental oxygen can decrease $D_{L_{CO}}$ by increasing the oxyhemoglobin

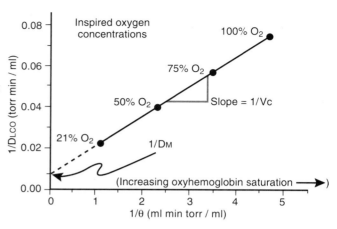

Figure 6–11. Measurement of D_M and V_C. If the diffusing capacity is measured while different concentrations of oxygen are being breathed, the value of $D_{L_{CO}}$ obtained will differ because the value of θ changes with the average hemoglobin saturation. When $1/D_{L_{CO}}$ is plotted against $1/\theta$, a straight line is obtained. The intercept of this line with the ordinate defines the membrane component of the resistance to gas transfer $(1/D_M)$, and the slope of the line varies inversely with the pulmonary capillary blood volume $(1/V_C)$.

saturation, thereby decreasing the value of θ. By increasing the carboxyhemoglobin content of blood (and thus blood P_{CO}), cigarette smoking can also decrease the measurement of $D_{L_{CO}}$.

E X A M P L E. A patient inhales a breath of air containing 0.3% carbon monoxide from residual volume to TLC and holds his breath for 10 seconds. Measuring the concentration of carbon monoxide during exhalation indicates that the average alveolar P_{CO} was 0.1 torr and that 0.67 ml of carbon monoxide was taken up during that time. What is the diffusing capacity for carbon monoxide? Since the blood P_{CO} is assumed to remain at zero, the average ΔP between blood and alveolar gas is 0.1 torr. For this ΔP, about 4.0 ml/min would be absorbed, so

$$D_{L_{CO}} = 40 \; \frac{ml/min}{torr}.$$ ∎

E X A M P L E. Plot the values of $1/D_{L_{CO}}$ that would be found if it were measured at different levels of $1/\theta$ (as defined in equation 5).

Figure 6–11 shows the relationship between $1/\theta$ and $1/D_{L_{CO}}$ as a straight line of the form $y = a + bx$. In this form, the slope of the line is $1/V_C$ and the y-intercept is the value $1/D_M$. Clinically, sequential $D_{L_{CO}}$ measurements are made as the subject breathes different concentrations of inspired oxygen. The values of $D_{L_{CO}}$ measured will therefore change because the average oxygen saturation in the pulmonary capillaries changes, thus varying θ. Extrapolating the line formed by the measurements to the ordinate gives the $D_{L_{CO}}$ value that would be found if the $1/(\theta V_C)$ resistance term were zero (i.e., if all the resistance to uptake had been in the membrane). Normally, about half of the resistance to gas uptake arises from the membrane resistance term $(1/D_M)$ and the remaining half from the resistance offered by the plasma and hemoglobin uptake term $(1/(\theta V_C))$. ∎

Chapter 7

Ventilation– Perfusion Relationships

For diffusion of gases to occur across the alveolar blood-gas barrier, a partial pressure difference must exist between alveolar gas and the blood entering the capillaries. As gas exchange occurs, this partial pressure gradient is maintained by alveolar ventilation and continued blood flow. Without blood flow, any blood remaining in the capillaries would quickly equilibrate with alveolar gas. Likewise, without ventilation the alveolar gas would quickly equilibrate with mixed venous blood and gas exchange would cease as the partial pressure gradients disappeared.

The ventilation–perfusion ratio is defined as the ratio of ventilation to blood flow for a single alveolus, a group of alveoli, or even the entire lung. For a single alveolus, this would be its ventilation ($\dot{V}_A$) divided by its capillary blood flow ($\dot{Q}$). For the whole lung, the ventilation–perfusion ratio is the total alveolar ventilation ($\dot{V}_A$) divided by the entire pulmonary blood flow ($\dot{Q}t$, cardiac output). Hence, a resting adult with an alveolar ventilation of 5 liters/min and a cardiac output of 5 liters/min would have an overall ventilation–perfusion ratio of about 1.0. Note that because ventilation and blood flow are expressed in the same units, this is a dimensionless parameter. The overall ventilation–perfusion ratio says little about the gas exchange function of the lung. For example, consider the situation that would occur if the 250 million to 300 million alveoli in the lung were numbered sequentially. If only the "even numbered" alveoli in a lung received blood flow and if only the "odd numbered" alveoli received any ventilation, then no gas exchange would take place even though the overall $\dot{V}_A/\dot{Q}$ ratio would be normal!

This chapter focuses on the effects of ventilation and blood flow on gas exchange in the lung. This is approached by first considering how ventilation and blood flow in a single alveolus influence its gas exchange. Next, the behavior of a whole lung consisting of many alveoli with identical ventilation and perfusion is considered. The situation that occurs when the lung is composed of two or more subpopulations of alveoli, each with a different ratio of blood flow to perfusion, is considered next. Finally, the case when the lungs are composed of many groups of alveoli with differing $\dot{V}_A/\dot{Q}$ ratios is described. When discussing the partial pressures in gas or blood, note that it is common to use "A" to denote alveolar gas, "a" to denote arterial blood, "$\overline{v}$" to denote mixed venous blood, and "ɪ" to refer to inspired gas.

VENTILATION–PERFUSION RATIO IN A SINGLE ALVEOLUS

Under normal circumstances, the rate of equilibration for oxygen and carbon dioxide along the pulmonary capillary is rapid enough to ensure that blood exiting from the end of a capillary has the same P_{O_2} and P_{CO_2} as its alveolar gas. Thus, the exchange of these gases is perfusion limited (see Chapter 6). In any single alveolus, the most important factor influencing the alveolar P_{O_2} and P_{CO_2} is the ratio of ventilation to perfusion ($\dot{V}_A/\dot{Q}$). Since the P_{O_2} and P_{CO_2} of blood exiting from the end of the alveolar capillary determine the respective blood oxygen and carbon dioxide contents, the $\dot{V}_A/\dot{Q}$ ratio of an alveolus is the major determinant of the end-capillary blood oxygen and carbon dioxide contents. To understand this better, consider a single alveolus as if it were a mixing tank, as shown in Figure 7–1. Here, cold water (analogous to mixed venous blood) is pumped into the tank through the pipe and hot water (analogous to alveolar ventila-

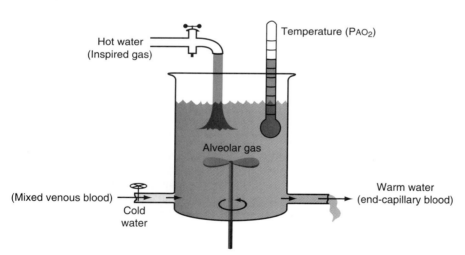

Figure 7–1. Effect of the ventilation–perfusion ratio on the alveolar gas composition in a single alveolus in the lung. Each alveolus behaves like a mixing tank, where the alveolar P_{O_2} is analogous to the temperature of the water in the tank. Hot water pours in at the top (analogous to alveolar ventilation), and cold water is pumped in at the bottom (analogous to mixed venous blood flow). The temperature of the hot water supply is analogous to the inspired P_{O_2}, and the temperature of the cold water supply is analogous to the mixed venous blood P_{O_2}. The P_{O_2} in an alveolus is determined by the balance between ventilation (hot water flow) and perfusion (cold water flow). Note that for any given $\dot{V}_A/\dot{Q}$ ratio, the alveolar P_{O_2} (water temperature in the tank) will also be influenced by the inspired and mixed venous P_{O_2} (temperatures of hot and cold water supplies).

tion) flows in at the top. In this analogy, the temperatures of the hot and cold water supplies are analogous to the inspired gas and mixed venous oxygen tensions ($P\bar{v}_{O_2}$ and $P_{I_{O_2}}$), while the flow rates are analogous to ventilation and blood flow rates. The temperature of the mixture in the tank is analogous to the P_{O_2} in alveolar gas. Obviously, the temperature in the tank represents a balance between how fast the hot and cold water sources are flowing (the ventilation-to-blood flow ratio) and the temperatures of the hot and cold water supplies (inspired P_{O_2} and mixed venous blood P_{O_2}, respectively). Note that the water leaving the system (analogous to end-capillary blood) has the same temperature (P_{O_2}) as the water in the tank (alveolar gas P_{O_2}). When the hot water and cold water flow rates are about equal, the water exiting from the tank (alveolus) is warm (normal alveolar $P_{O_2} = 100$ torr). If the "$\dot{V}_A/\dot{Q}$ ratio" of the tank is decreased by lowering the inflow rate of hot water (decreasing alveolar ventilation), then the temperature of water in the tank (alveolar P_{O_2}) will decrease toward the cold water supply temperature (mixed venous P_{O_2}). Conversely, if the $\dot{V}_A/\dot{Q}$ ratio is increased by decreasing the flow rate of cold water (or by increasing the flow of hot water), the temperature in the tank will increase toward the hot water supply temperature (alveolar P_{O_2} will increase toward inspired P_{O_2}). Note that if the hot water flow is turned off entirely, the "$\dot{V}_A/\dot{Q}$ ratio" of the tank will decrease to zero, and the temperature in the tank will eventually decrease to equal that of the cold water supply (mixed venous P_{O_2}). Thus, the P_{O_2} in an alveolus with $\dot{V}_A/\dot{Q}$ ratio of zero will eventually decrease only to the P_{O_2} in mixed venous blood. On the other hand, if the $\dot{V}_A/\dot{Q}$ ratio of the tank is increased (by decreasing the cold water flow or increasing the hot water flow), the temperature will increase toward the hot water supply temperature. Thus, an alveolus with an infinite $\dot{V}_A/\dot{Q}$ ratio (some ventilation but no blood flow) will have an alveolar P_{O_2} equal to the inspired gas P_{O_2}. From this, it should be clear that the P_{O_2} in any single alveolus must lie somewhere between the mixed venous P_{O_2} and the inspired P_{O_2}, depending on what its $\dot{V}_A/\dot{Q}$ ratio is.

A similar analysis can be applied to carbon dioxide. Normally, there is virtually no carbon dioxide in inspired gas because the atmospheric P_{CO_2} is only about 0.2 torr. Thus, the P_{CO_2} in any single alveolus

depends on the P_{CO_2} in mixed venous blood (normally about 47 torr) and the $\dot{V}_A/\dot{Q}$ ratio of the alveolus. Normally, the alveolar P_{CO_2} and end-capillary blood P_{CO_2} are in equilibrium (perfusion-limited exchange). When breathing air, the alveolar gas and end-capillary blood in a single alveolus will have a P_{CO_2} that lies somewhere between mixed venous P_{CO_2} and zero. If the $\dot{V}_A/\dot{Q}$ ratio is close to zero, the alveolar P_{CO_2} will approach the mixed venous P_{CO_2}. As the $\dot{V}_A/\dot{Q}$ ratio in an alveolus is increased, the alveolar P_{CO_2} decreases, until it equals the inspired P_{CO_2} (normally zero) in an alveolus with infinite $\dot{V}_A/\dot{Q}$ ratio (i.e., ventilation but no blood flow).

VENTILATION–PERFUSION RATIOS IN A LUNG WITH IDENTICAL ALVEOLI

Oxygen Exchange

Consider what would happen if all the alveoli in the lungs had the same $\dot{V}_A/\dot{Q}$ ratio. This is a purely hypothetical situation, since not all alveoli have the same $\dot{V}_A/\dot{Q}$ ratio even in healthy lungs. Since the inspired gas P_{O_2} and the mixed venous blood P_{O_2} are normally the same for every alveolus, the alveolar P_{O_2} would be identical in every alveolus (assuming that they all had the same $\dot{V}_A/\dot{Q}$ ratio). The end-capillary blood P_{O_2} and content values would also be identical for every alveolus because the blood exiting from each alveolus has a P_{O_2} equal to that in its alveolar gas. Consequently, the systemic arterial blood P_{O_2} would be equal to the P_{O_2} within each alveolus, because systemic arterial blood is a mixture of end-capillary blood from all of the alveoli. Likewise, the alveolar P_{CO_2} would be the same in every alveolus, and the arterial blood would have the same P_{CO_2} as present in alveolar gas. In this situation the lung is said to be *homogeneous* with respect to its $\dot{V}_A/\dot{Q}$ ratios.

An equivalent way of describing such a *homogeneous lung* would be to represent the whole lung as if it were a single giant alveolus, with a blood flow equal to the cardiac output, and an alveolar ventilation equal to the total alveolar ventilation (Figure 7–2). The gas exchange behavior of a homogeneous lung can be thought of as *ideal,* in the sense that the arterial blood P_{O_2} and P_{CO_2} values it yields are iden-

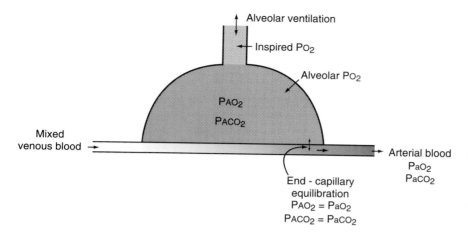

Figure 7-2. The *ideal lung* represented as a single alveolus. When all alveoli in a lung have the same ratio of ventilation to blood flow, the lung is homogeneous with respect to $\dot{V}_A/\dot{Q}$. In this ideal situation, the lung can be represented as if it were a single large alveolus receiving all the blood flow and all of the ventilation. This is an ideal lung because the arterial blood leaving it has the same P_{aO_2} and P_{aCO_2} as the ideal alveolar gas (P_{AO_2} and P_{ACO_2}). Thus, the $(A - a)D_{O_2}$ for this lung would be zero.

tical to the alveolar gas P_{O_2} and P_{CO_2}. The alveolar P_{O_2} (P_{AO_2}) in an ideal lung such as this can be calculated using the *ideal alveolar oxygen equation:*

$$P_{AO_2} = P_{IO_2} - \frac{P_{ACO_2}}{R} \text{ or}$$

$$P_{AO_2} = F_{IO_2} \cdot (P_{baro} - 47) - \frac{P_{ACO_2}}{R}$$

where F_{IO_2} is the inspired oxygen fraction (i.e., percentage divided by 100), P_{IO_2} is the inspired oxygen tension [$P_{IO_2} = (P_{baro} - 47) F_{IO_2}$], P_{ACO_2} is the alveolar gas carbon dioxide tension, P_{baro} is the ambient barometric pressure, and R is the *respiratory exchange ratio*. The respiratory exchange ratio is the ratio of carbon dioxide excreted ($\dot{V}_{CO_2}$) relative to the oxygen taken up ($\dot{V}_{O_2}$) by the lungs:

$$R = \frac{\dot{V}_{CO_2}}{\dot{V}_{O_2}}$$

In steady state, R is equal to the *metabolic respiratory quotient* (RQ), defined as the number of carbon dioxide molecules produced relative to oxygen molecules consumed by intermediary metabolism. In a subject in normal nutritional status, RQ (and thus R) usually lies between 0.7 and 1.0, depending on the balance of fatty acids and carbohydrates used as energetic substrates for metabolism. If fatty acids are metabolized exclusively by the body, the RQ would be about 0.7, whereas an RQ of 1.0 would occur if carbohydrate was used exclusively for

steady-state energy production (see Chapter 9). Note that when R is less than 1.0, the volume of gas exhaled over time will be slightly less than the inhaled volume, because more oxygen is taken up than carbon dioxide released in the alveoli.

EXAMPLE. What is the ideal alveolar P_{O_2} in a subject breathing a 50% oxygen mixture if the respiratory exchange ratio is 0.85 and the arterial P_{CO_2} is 40 torr?

Here, the inspired oxygen tension (P_{IO_2}) equals the ambient barometric pressure ($P_{baro} = 760$ torr at sea level) minus the water vapor tension (47 torr) times the inspired oxygen fraction ($F_{IO_2} = 0.5$). In general, the arterial P_{CO_2} (P_{aCO_2}) is about the same as the alveolar P_{CO_2} (P_{ACO_2}). Thus,

$$P_{AO_2} = 356.5 - 47.1 = 309.4 \text{ torr.} \quad \blacksquare$$

The oxygen tension in alveolar gas is less than inspired P_{O_2} because it reflects a balance between the rate that oxygen is delivered to the alveoli and the rate that it is taken up into alveolar capillary blood. The delivery of oxygen into the alveoli depends on the inspired ventilation and the inspired P_{O_2}. The rate that oxygen is taken up into blood is determined by the oxygen needs of the tissues ($\dot{V}_{O_2}$). Thus, if the inspired P_{O_2} is increased while the metabolic rate ($\dot{V}_{O_2}$) stays constant, the alveolar P_{O_2} will increase. Conversely, if the minute ventilation and P_{IO_2} are held constant while the subject exercises, the alveolar P_{O_2} will decrease. This is not immediately apparent from the alveolar oxygen equation above, because the $\dot{V}O_2$ and the inspired and exhaled ventilation terms have been algebraically eliminated. Nevertheless, the PIO_2 term reflects the rate that oxygen is delivered to the alveoli, and the $PACO_2/R$ term represents the rate that oxygen leaves the alveolus as it is taken up into blood. Recall that the sum of all gas partial pressures in the alveoli must equal the total pressure. When breathing air, alveolar gas contains oxygen, carbon dioxide, water vapor, nitrogen, and trace amounts of inert gases such as argon. When breathing pure oxygen, the only gases present in the alveoli are oxygen, carbon dioxide, and water. Note that if a subject breathes pure oxygen, the alveolar PO_2 is simply the $PIO_2 - PH_2O - PACO_2$, because these are the only gases present in the alveolus.

The alveolar PO_2 calculated using the ideal alveolar gas equation represents the greatest *arterial* PO_2 that such a lung could produce. Thus, when the arterial PO_2 (PaO_2) is equal to the PAO_2 calculated using this equation, the lung is operating at its highest efficiency as a gas exchanger. It would be impossible for the PaO_2 to be any greater without either increasing the inflowing concentration of oxygen (PIO_2) or decreasing the rate that oxygen is taken out of the alveoli into blood ($PACO_2/R$). Thus, in the ideal lung the *alveolar-arterial PO_2 difference* is zero:

Alveolar–arterial PO_2 difference $[(A - a)DO_2]$

$= $ Ideal alveolar PO_2 − measured PaO_2

The calculated $(A - a)DO_2$ provides an approximate measure of how well the lung is acting as a gas exchanger. In general, the larger the $(A - a)DO_2$, the worse the efficiency of gas exchange. This concept becomes more important in later sections dealing with ventilation–perfusion inequality in nonhomogeneous lungs.

Carbon Dioxide Exchange

Recall from Chapter 3 that the PCO_2 in alveolar gas reflects a balance between the rate that carbon dioxide enters alveolar gas from blood ($\dot{V}CO_2$, ml/min) and the rate that alveolar ventilation ($\dot{V}A$, ml/min) washes it out. Because inspired gas normally contains no carbon dioxide, the product of alveolar ventilation ($\dot{V}A$) and the fraction of $\dot{V}A$ that is carbon

dioxide must equal the exhaled flow of carbon dioxide ($\dot{V}CO_2$):

$$\dot{V}CO_2 = \dot{V}A \cdot FACO_2$$

This equation can be solved for the alveolar carbon dioxide tension ($PACO_2$), since

$$PACO_2 = FACO_2 \cdot (P_{baro} - PH_2O):$$

Thus,

$$PACO_2 = \frac{\dot{V}CO_2(P_{baro} - PH_2O)}{\dot{V}A}$$

This is the *ideal alveolar gas equation for carbon dioxide.* It says that the alveolar PCO_2 is set by the ratio of carbon dioxide production to the alveolar ventilation. Because $PaCO_2$ is same as the $PACO_2$ in the ideal lung (see Figure 7–2), $PaCO_2$ is set by the level of alveolar ventilation relative to the level of metabolic activity.

E X A M P L E. A comatose patient arrives at the emergency department of a hospital. Among other tests, an arterial blood sample is drawn from the radial artery. Analysis of the sample in a *blood gas analyzer* yields $PaO_2 = 46$ torr and $PaCO_2 = 85$ torr. Why is the patient's PaO_2 abnormally low?

First, calculate the ideal alveolar PO_2 to find out how high the arterial PO_2 ought to be if the lung were operating ideally. Assuming an $R = 0.85$, then the ideal alveolar oxygen equation would be

$$PAO_2 = PIO_2 - PACO_2/0.85$$

Since the barometric pressure is 760 torr and the patient is at 37°C,

$$PIO_2 = (760 - 47)\, 0.209 = 149 \text{ torr}$$

Assume that the $PaCO_2$ is the same as the $PACO_2$. Thus,

$$PAO_2 = 149 - 85/0.85 = 49 \text{ torr}$$

$$(A - a)DO_2 = 49 - 46 = 3 \text{ torr}$$

Thus, the greatest PaO_2 that could be expected in

this patient is only 49 torr; the measured P_{aO_2} is only 3 torr less than this. Therefore the low arterial P_{O_2} (*hypoxemia*) is caused by a low alveolar P_{O_2}. Note that the high alveolar P_{CO_2} in this case (relative to a normal P_{CO_2} of 40 torr) is caused by inadequate alveolar ventilation. The low alveolar P_{O_2} is also the result of inadequate alveolar ventilation. Inadequate alveolar ventilation has reduced the alveolar P_{O_2} by reducing the rate of oxygen inflow into the lung, relative to its rate of uptake into blood. In this patient, the decreased alveolar ventilation was initially caused by a depressed ventilatory drive arising from an overdose of barbiturates, which depress ventilation. This patient was treated by use of mechanical ventilation, applied through an endotracheal tube positioned in the trachea. Restoration of normal alveolar ventilation caused the arterial P_{CO_2} to decrease to 38 torr and the arterial P_{O_2} to increase to 97 torr. ■

GAS EXCHANGE IN NONIDEAL LUNGS: THE EFFECTS OF VENTILATION – PERFUSION INEQUALITY

In healthy lungs the $\dot{V}_A/\dot{Q}$ ratios of all alveoli are not equal. Recall (see Chapter 1) that alveoli near the top of a vertical lung are less well ventilated than alveoli near the bottom, owing to the effects of gravity on the distribution of pleural (and transpulmonary) pressures. Likewise, alveoli near the top of the lung receive less blood flow than those near the base, because of the effects of gravity on the pulmonary circulation (see Chapter 4). Because the decrease in blood flow from the top to the bottom of the lung is more marked than the decrease in ventilation, the ratio of $\dot{V}_A/\dot{Q}$ is also different in alveoli in different regions of the lung. The presence of alveoli with widely different $\dot{V}_A/\dot{Q}$ ratios in a lung reduces the overall efficiency of gas exchange by the lung.

In many forms of lung disease, nonuniform changes in the mechanical properties of the lungs or the pulmonary circulation can cause dramatic increases in the disparity of $\dot{V}_A/\dot{Q}$ ratios among alveoli. For example, diseased lungs may have $\dot{V}_A/\dot{Q}$ ratios that differ among alveoli by a factor of 1,000 or more. This can reduce dramatically the efficiency of lung gas exchange and contribute to severe arterial hypoxemia.

The extent to which the $\dot{V}_A/\dot{Q}$ ratios differ among alveoli is referred to as *the degree of ventilation–perfusion inequality*. Even though the overall $\dot{V}_A/\dot{Q}$ ratio for the lung remains in the normal range, an individual alveolus may have a $\dot{V}_A/\dot{Q}$ ratio very different from this because of changes in either its ventilation or blood flow. When some alveoli in the lung have different $\dot{V}_A/\dot{Q}$ ratios from others, gas exchange occurs less efficiently than if all the alveoli are alike in their ratio of ventilation to blood flow. This decrease in efficiency causes an increase in the $(A-a)D_{O_2}$ by reducing the arterial P_{O_2}.

The Two-Compartment Lung

To understand how ventilation–perfusion inequality interferes with gas exchange, consider a lung composed of two subpopulations of alveoli, as shown in Figure 7–3. The cardiac output is 5 liters/min and the alveolar ventilation is 5 liters/min, so the overall $\dot{V}_A/\dot{Q}$ ratio for the lung is 1.0. One group of alveoli receives 80% of the cardiac output (4 liters/min) and 98% of the alveolar ventilation (4.9 liters/min); its $\dot{V}_A/\dot{Q}$ ratio would be about 1.2. For this example, assume that this first group is homogeneous; that is, each alveolus in it has a $\dot{V}_A/\dot{Q}$ ratio of 1.2. A second subpopulation of alveoli receives 20% of the blood flow (1.0 liter/min) and 2% of the ventilation (0.1 liter/min). Its $\dot{V}_A/\dot{Q}$ ratio is low (0.1) because ventilation has been partially obstructed by a mucus plug in a bronchus. Once again, assume that these alveoli all have the same low $\dot{V}_A/\dot{Q}$ ratio. Because the $\dot{V}_A/\dot{Q}$ ratio of the second group is decreased, these alveoli will exhibit an alveolar P_{O_2} that is closer to the $P_{\bar{v}O_2}$ (35.5 torr) than the first group. By virtue of their relatively higher $\dot{V}_A/\dot{Q}$ ratio, the alveolar P_{O_2} in the first group will be greater than in the second group.

In this example, the P_{aO_2} in the high $\dot{V}_A/\dot{Q}$ group is 113 torr, while that in the low $\dot{V}_A/\dot{Q}$ group is 42 torr. [Note that this is not a trivial calculation, since the R values in the two compartments will not be the same as the overall R for the lung!] Thus, blood exiting from alveoli in the high $\dot{V}_A/\dot{Q}$ population will have a P_{O_2} of 113 torr; the hemoglobin therefore will be about 98% saturated with oxygen. Blood exiting from alveoli in the low $\dot{V}_A/\dot{Q}$ compartment will have a P_{O_2} of 42 torr, which corresponds to a hemoglobin saturation of 74%. The mixture of these therefore will be 93.2% saturated

Figure 7–3. A lung composed of two functional subpopulations of alveoli. The $\dot{V}_A/\dot{Q}$ ratio is the same for all alveoli within each group, but is different between groups. One group of alveoli ($\dot{V}_A/\dot{Q}$ = 1.2) receives a blood flow of 4 liters/min and an alveolar ventilation of 4.9 liters/min. The second group ($\dot{V}_A/\dot{Q}$ = 0.1) receives a blood flow of 1.0 liter/min and an alveolar ventilation of 0.1 liter/min. Because their $\dot{V}_A/\dot{Q}$ ratio is higher, the first group will have an alveolar P_{O_2} closer to the inspired P_{O_2}, while the second group has an alveolar P_{O_2} closer to mixed venous P_{O_2}. End-capillary blood exiting from the two populations combines to form systemic arterial blood, with Pa_{O_2} = 67 torr and Pa_{CO_2} = 37 torr. Note that the systemic arterial blood oxygen *content* represents a blood flow-weighted average of the oxygen *contents* exiting from the two populations of alveoli.

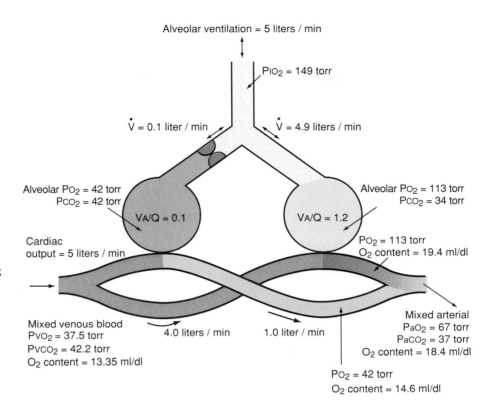

Alveolar ventilation = 5 liters / min

P_{IO_2} = 149 torr

$\dot{V}$ = 0.1 liter / min $\dot{V}$ = 4.9 liters / min

Alveolar P_{O_2} = 42 torr
P_{CO_2} = 42 torr

$\dot{V}_A/\dot{Q}$ = 0.1

Alveolar P_{O_2} = 113 torr
P_{CO_2} = 34 torr

$\dot{V}_A/\dot{Q}$ = 1.2

Cardiac output = 5 liters / min

P_{O_2} = 113 torr
O_2 content = 19.4 ml/dl

Mixed venous blood
P_{VO_2} = 37.5 torr
P_{VCO_2} = 42.2 torr
O_2 content = 13.35 ml/dl

4.0 liters / min   1.0 liter / min

Mixed arterial
Pa_{O_2} = 67 torr
Pa_{CO_2} = 37 torr
O_2 content = 18.4 ml/dl

P_{O_2} = 42 torr
O_2 content = 14.6 ml/dl

with oxygen (80% of the blood flow at 98% saturation + 20% of the blood flow at 74% saturation). Figure 7–4 shows how blood from the two subpopulations combines to form systemic arterial blood. Blood from the high $\dot{V}_A/\dot{Q}$ group (4 liters/min) is 98% saturated and has an oxygen content of 19.4 ml/dl. Blood from the low $\dot{V}_A/\dot{Q}$ region (1 liter/min) is 74% saturated and has an oxygen content of 14.6 ml/dl. The arterial mixture of these has an oxygen content of 18.4 ml/dl and a saturation of about 93%. From the dissociation curve shown in Figure 7–4, this corresponds with a P_{O_2} of 67 torr. Note that the arterial oxygen content reflects a flow-weighted contribution from the end-capillary oxygen contents of the two populations of alveoli. The P_{O_2} in systemic arterial blood is that value corresponding to the oxygen saturation of the arterial mixture and not merely a numerical average of the end-capillary P_{O_2} values.

The ideal alveolar P_{O_2} can be calculated for the above example using the alveolar oxygen equation. If the Pa_{CO_2} = 40 torr and the respiratory exchange

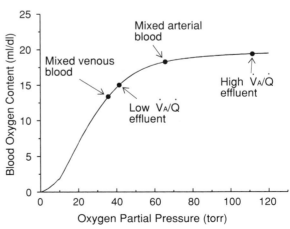

Figure 7–4. Relationship between P_{O_2} and oxygen content in blood. The blood oxygen contents exiting from the two subpopulations of alveoli (shown in Figure 7–3) are shown, along with the composition of systemic arterial blood.

ratio of 0.85 is assumed, then

$$P_{AO_2} = (760 - 47) \cdot 0.209 - \frac{40}{0.85} = 102 \text{ torr}$$

This is the alveolar P_{O_2} that would have been found if the lung were homogeneous. Note that there are no alveoli in the lung that actually have this P_{AO_2}. The $(A - a)D_{O_2}$ for this lung would therefore be 102 − 67 = 35 torr. This means that the blood leaving this lung has a P_{O_2} that is 35 torr less than it would have been with no ventilation–perfusion inequality.

VENTILATION–PERFUSION INEQUALITY IN MULTICOMPARTMENT LUNG MODELS

It is theoretically possible for each of the approximately 300 million alveoli to have a unique $\dot{V}_A/\dot{Q}$ ratio, which could range from zero (for an alveolus with no ventilation) to infinity (for one with no perfusion). Obviously, analyzing the behavior of a lung would be a complex process if each alveolus is considered separately. It turns out that an excellent approximation of any real lung can be made if alveoli are partitioned into eight or more potential separate populations (compartments), each characterized by a unique value of $\dot{V}_A/\dot{Q}$. Thus, each compartment consists of all the alveoli whose $\dot{V}_A/\dot{Q}$ ratios are nearest that value. A logarithmic scale of $\dot{V}_A/\dot{Q}$ ratios is chosen to span the physiological range of potential $\dot{V}_A/\dot{Q}$ ratios. Figure 7–5A shows such a lung model, with compartment $\dot{V}_A/\dot{Q}$ ratios ranging from zero to infinity. These should be thought of as potential compartments because a given lung may or may not have alveoli with all of these values. Thus, to describe a particular lung, one must partition the blood flow and ventilation for each alveolus into the compartment that most closely resembles its operating $\dot{V}_A/\dot{Q}$ ratio.

For example, the histogram shown in Figure 7–5B describes the distribution of blood flow and ventilation in a relatively healthy lung. Note that about 90% of the blood flow through this lung travels through alveoli whose $\dot{V}_A/\dot{Q}$ ratios are nearly identical. About 5% of the blood flow is distributed to alveoli with $\dot{V}_A/\dot{Q}$ ratios tenfold lower, and about 5% is distributed to alveoli with $\dot{V}_A/\dot{Q}$ ratios about tenfold greater than the major mode (which hap-

pens to reside at a $\dot{V}_A/\dot{Q}$ near unity). No alveoli in a normal lung should have $\dot{V}_A/\dot{Q}$ ratios of 0.01 or 0.001 or 0.0, and none occur in this lung. Likewise, there are no alveoli in this lung with $\dot{V}_A/\dot{Q}$ ratios of 100. Note that alveoli with a $\dot{V}_A/\dot{Q}$ ratio of infinity (i.e., alveolar dead space) could be present in this lung, but they would not be apparent from the blood flow distribution (Figure 7–5B) because their blood flows would always be zero. For this reason, it is common to show both the distribution of blood flow and the distribution of ventilation in such a model.

Figure 7–6 shows the distribution of blood flow and the distribution of ventilation in a multi-compartment lung model. As in Figure 7–5B, this distribution is characteristic of a normal lung. Gas exchange would be relatively efficient in this lung, because it is nearly homogeneous, that is, most of the alveoli have nearly the same $\dot{V}_A/\dot{Q}$ ratio. Thus, this lung behaves much like the single-compartment lung described earlier, and its $(A - a)D_{O_2}$ will be relatively small. Experimental measurements of the $\dot{V}_A/\dot{Q}$ distribution in normal subjects yield results similar to that shown in Figure 7–6.

In contrast to the lung shown in Figure 7–6, the $\dot{V}_A/\dot{Q}$ distribution shown in Figure 7–7 is highly abnormal. This lung has the same blood flow and alveolar ventilation as the example shown in Figure 7–6, but the distribution is far more heterogeneous with respect to $\dot{V}_A/\dot{Q}$ dispersion. Note that more than 20% of the cardiac output perfuses alveoli with $\dot{V}_A/\dot{Q}$ less then 0.1, and much of the ventilation is distributed to alveoli that receive less than 10% of the blood flow ($\dot{V}_A/\dot{Q}$ greater than 10). By virtue of their differing $\dot{V}_A/\dot{Q}$ ratios, alveoli among different compartments will have widely varying alveolar P_{O_2} values. Accordingly, the end-capillary hemoglobin oxygen saturations (and blood oxygen contents) will also vary widely among compartments. In the lung shown in Figure 7–7, the systemic arterial blood would have an oxygen saturation (reflecting the flow-weighted average of blood oxygen contents from each compartment) of only 75%, corresponding to an arterial P_{O_2} of 45 torr. For this lung, the ideal alveolar P_{O_2} can be calculated using the alveolar oxygen equation, yielding an ideal P_{AO_2} = 98.8 torr. Thus, the $\dot{V}_A/\dot{Q}$ heterogeneity present in this lung has given rise to a large increase in the $(A - a)D_{O_2}$ and a reduction in the efficiency of gas exchange.

Figure 7–5. *A.* A multi-compartment lung model, allowing for the possible existence of alveoli with widely varying V̇A/Q̇. With the use of this model, a relatively normal lung is described by the histogram. Note that there are no alveoli in this normal lung with V̇A/Q̇ less than 0.1. Most of the blood flow is distributed to alveoli with nearly the same V̇A/Q̇, which happens to lie near 1.0. Only small amounts of blood flow are distributed to alveoli with V̇A/Q̇ near 0.1 or 10.0 . Hence, most of the "potential compartments" are unused in this example. *B.* A relatively homogeneous lung. This histogram describes how much blood flow travels to alveoli with V̇A/Q̇ ratios corresponding to the compartment values. Note that most of the blood flow is distributed to alveoli with nearly the same V̇A/Q̇ ratio.

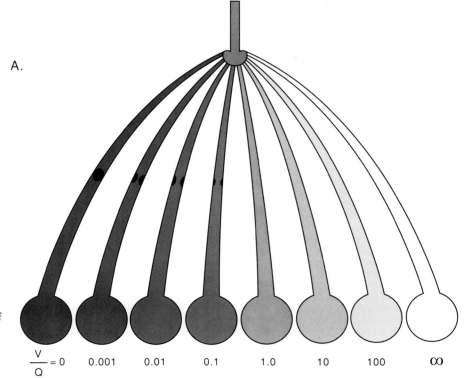

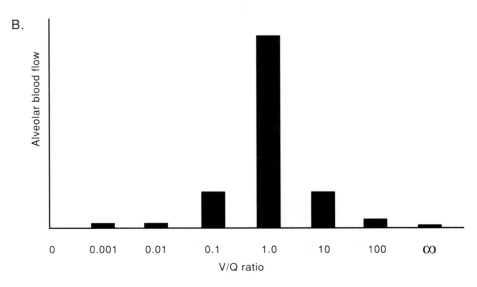

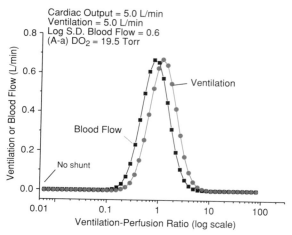

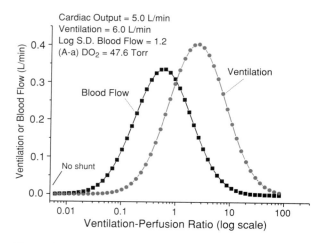

Figure 7-6. Ventilation and perfusion distributed in a multicompartment lung model. Points along the "blood flow" curve represent a histogram, showing the amount of blood flow passing through alveolar compartments with the corresponding $\dot{V}_A/\dot{Q}$ ratio. Points along the "ventilation" curve show the amount of ventilation going to alveoli with that $\dot{V}_A/\dot{Q}$ ratio. Although this lung is not homogeneous, most of the blood flow and ventilation are distributed to alveoli with nearly the same $\dot{V}_A/\dot{Q}$ ratio. Hence, the (A − a)Do$_2$ for this lung will be relatively small. Note that the sum of compartmental blood flows must equal cardiac output and that the ventilations must sum to equal total alveolar ventilation. Note also that if the blood flow to a given $\dot{V}_A/\dot{Q}$ compartment is known, the corresponding ventilation can be calculated.

Figure 7-7. Ventilation–perfusion distribution in a highly nonhomogeneous lung. Different alveoli within this lung exhibit $\dot{V}_A/\dot{Q}$ ratios ranging from less than 0.01 to more than 50. Because the alveolar Po$_2$ differs markedly among alveoli with different $\dot{V}_A/\dot{Q}$, the end-capillary blood oxygen saturations and contents will also differ among compartments. This lung exhibits an (A − a) Do$_2$ of about 48 torr.

Why is gas exchange less efficient in a lung with $\dot{V}_A/\dot{Q}$ heterogeneity? Much of the problem relates to the nonlinearity of the partial pressure–oxygen content relationship for blood. Poorly ventilated alveoli (i.e., those with low $\dot{V}_A/\dot{Q}$ ratios) have relatively low alveolar oxygen tensions as a result. Hence, blood leaving them has a relatively low oxygen content because the hemoglobin saturation is incomplete. Normal alveoli with $\dot{V}_A/\dot{Q}$ ratios between about 0.3 and 10 have alveolar oxygen tensions high enough so that blood leaving them is virtually fully saturated. Alveoli with high $\dot{V}_A/\dot{Q}$ ratios (greater than 10) have alveolar oxygen tensions that approach the inspired Po$_2$. However, this normally adds little additional oxygen content to the blood leaving them because only dissolved oxygen can be added. Therefore, overventilating some alveoli cannot compensate for the low oxygen content coming from poorly ventilated alveoli.

PULMONARY SHUNTING: AN EXTREME CASE OF VENTILATION–PERFUSION INEQUALITY

When some alveoli receive blood flow but are not ventilated, their alveolar (and end-capillary) Po$_2$ is the same as in mixed venous blood. This situation occurs in *pulmonary alveolar edema* when edema fluid fills the airspaces, preventing ventilation from reaching the alveolar-capillary membrane. Nonventilated alveoli can also develop if a bronchus is completely obstructed by mucus or other material, thereby preventing ventilation of some alveoli, or when a portion of the lung collapses (*atelectasis*), as may occur if large amounts of air enter the pleural space during *pneumothorax*. Regardless of the cause, continued blood flow through unventilated alveoli (*intrapulmonary shunting*) causes a fall in arterial Po$_2$ because desaturated blood (with the composition of mixed venous blood) exiting from nonventilated alveoli mixes with end-capillary blood from normally ventilated alveoli, thereby lowering the saturation of the mixture. Thus, shunting may be thought of as an extreme case of ventilation–perfusion inequality.

Figure 7–8 shows a three-compartment model of

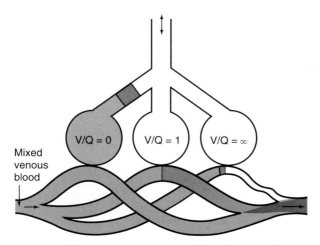

Figure 7–8. Three-compartment model of the lung, which allows for the existence of alveoli with blood flow but no ventilation ($\dot{V}A/\dot{Q} = 0$), normal blood flow and ventilation ($\dot{V}A/\dot{Q} \approx 1$), and ventilation but no blood flow ($\dot{V}A/\dot{Q} = \infty$). Note that all gas exchange in this lung occurs in the middle compartment.

the lung, which is a clinically useful model for describing the acute lung gas exchange disorders described earlier. This model is composed of three alveolar populations (or compartments) and is really a simplification of the multicompartment lung model shown in Figure 7–5A. The first compartment characterizes alveoli that receive blood flow but no ventilation ($\dot{V}A/\dot{Q} = 0$)—*the shunt compartment.* The second contains normally ventilated and perfused alveoli, analogous to the homogeneous *ideal* lung described above. The $\dot{V}A/\dot{Q}$ ratio in this group of alveoli is usually within the normal range of 0.3 to 10. The third population contains alveoli that receive ventilation but no blood flow ($\dot{V}A/\dot{Q} = \infty$). This model provides a good description of lungs with alveolar edema or atelectasis because the non-ventilated alveoli can be described by the shunt compartment, whereas the remainder of the alveoli (which are often normally ventilated and perfused) are described well by the middle compartment. As with the previous models, a particular lung is described by apportioning the relative blood flows to these compartments. Similarly, dead space ventilation can be described by apportioning some of the ventilation to the third compartment.

Clinically, it is often useful to be able to calculate the percentage of the cardiac output ($\dot{Q}_t$) passing through nonventilated alveoli (shunt), compared with normal alveoli. This is calculated simply if we know (1) $C\bar{v}o_2$: the oxygen content of mixed venous blood; (2) Cao_2: the oxygen content of arterial blood; and (3) $Cc'o_2$: the oxygen content of blood exiting from the normally ventilated and perfused compartment. Note that the flow of oxygen (ml/min) in arterial blood leaving the lung (cardiac output · Cao_2) must be the sum of the oxygen flow leaving the shunt alveoli (shunt blood flow · $C\bar{v}o_2$) and the oxygen flow leaving the normally ventilated alveoli (non-shunt flow · $Cc'o_2$):

$$\dot{Q}t \cdot Cao_2 = \dot{Q}s \cdot C\bar{v}o_2 + (\dot{Q}t - \dot{Q}s) \cdot Cc'o_2$$

This can be solved for the fraction of the cardiac output perfusing the shunt compartment:

$$\frac{\dot{Q}s}{\dot{Q}t} = \frac{Cc'o_2 - Cao_2}{Cc'o_2 - C\bar{v}o_2}$$

E X A M P L E. A patient breathing 100% oxygen has an arterial $Po_2 = 76$ torr, $Paco_2 = 40$ torr, and arterial oxygen saturation = 94.5%. Mixed venous blood $Po_2 = 35$ torr, with a hemoglobin saturation of 63%. The hemoglobin concentration is 14 g/dl. What is the shunt fraction in this patient?

First calculate the arterial oxygen content, as the sum of hemoglobin bound and dissolved oxygen components:

$$Cao_2 = 1.39 \text{ ml/g} \cdot 14 \text{ g/dl} \cdot 0.945 + 76 \text{ torr}$$

$$\cdot \ 0.003 \text{ ml/(dl torr)} = 18.62 \text{ ml/dl}$$

Next, calculate the mixed venous oxygen content:

$$C\bar{v}o_2 = 1.39 \text{ ml/g} \cdot 14 \text{ g/dl} \cdot 0.63 + 35 \text{ torr}$$

$$\cdot \ 0.003 \text{ ml/(dl torr)} = 12.37 \text{ ml/dl}$$

Finally, calculate the blood oxygen content exiting from the ideal compartment. This can be calculated if the alveolar Po_2 is determined using the ideal alveolar oxygen equation. When breathing pure oxygen, the ideal alveolar Po_2 is calculated by subtracting the water vapor and alveolar P_{CO_2} from the total barometric pressure (P_{baro}):

$$P_{AO_2} = P_{IO_2} - P_{ACO_2} - P_{H_2O}$$

$$P_{AO_2} = 760 - 40 - 47 = 673 \text{ torr}$$

Now, calculate the end-capillary ideal oxygen content (Cc'_{O_2}), assuming that hemoglobin with a P_{O_2} greater than 150 torr is 100% saturated:

$$Cc'_{O_2} = 1.39 \text{ ml/g} \cdot 14 \text{ g/dl} \cdot 1.0 + 673 \text{ torr} \cdot 0.003 \text{ ml/(dl torr)} = 21.48 \text{ ml/dl}$$

Now the shunt fraction can be calculated:

$$\frac{\dot{Q}s}{\dot{Q}t} = \frac{(21.48 - 18.62)}{(21.48 - 12.37)} = 0.31$$

Thus, about 69% of the cardiac output went to the ideal alveoli, while about 31% went to the shunt alveoli, thereby explaining the large $(A-a)D_{O_2}$ (673 − 76 = 597 torr). ■

Note that the oxygen shunt equation can be applied to any lung, regardless of whether any nonventilated alveoli ($\dot{V}A/\dot{Q} = 0$) are present. For example, the lung described in Figure 7–7 has no shunt, since all of its alveoli receive at least some ventilation. Yet application of the shunt equation to that lung yields a "shunt" value of 47%. This occurs because the three-compartment lung model (Figure 7–8) is inadequate to describe the lung shown in Figure 7–7, since it does not allow for the possible existence of ventilation–perfusion inequality. In this example, the shunt equation describes the lung of Figure 7–7 as if it contained shunt alveoli receiving 47% of the cardiac output. The normally ventilated and perfused alveoli receive 53% of the cardiac output. In other words, a homogeneous lung with the same mixed venous blood composition and inspired gas (as in Figure 7–7) would need a 47% shunt to have the same arterial P_{O_2} as seen for the lung in Figure 7–7. The "shunt" value calculated for a lung that has ventilation–perfusion inequality is termed the *venous admixture,* to acknowledge that the value is an "as if" shunt.

Extrapulmonary Shunting

All blood that travels through the pulmonary circulation must also pass through pulmonary alveolar capillaries because there are no pulmonary arteriovenous vessels that would allow blood flow to bypass the capillaries. In normal lungs, virtually all of the alveoli are open and ventilated and can exchange gas with capillary blood. Hence, there is virtually no shunting of blood flow in healthy lungs. However, under some circumstances blood flow may bypass the pulmonary circulation, thereby contributing mixed venous blood directly into the systemic arterial blood supply. This *extrapulmonary shunting* causes arterial hypoxemia by the same mechanism as nonventilated lung regions. For example, if the *ductus arteriosus* (see Chapter 10) fails to close after birth, or if a hole in the septal wall separating the left and right ventricles *(septal defect)* is present, mixed venous blood may enter the arterial system and cause arterial hypoxemia, even though the lungs are entirely normal. Another source of extrapulmonary shunting arises from *thebesian veins.* These veins drain a small portion of the coronary venous blood flow directly into the left ventricle, rather than into the coronary sinus in the right atrium. Although thebesian venous blood flow is small, the blood is highly desaturated and its addition to systemic arterial blood lowers its oxygen content slightly. Yet another source of extrapulmonary shunting arises from the *bronchial circulation.* The large airways and bronchi are nourished by systemic arterial blood through the bronchial circulation. A portion of the bronchial venous blood drains into the pulmonary circulation downstream from the alveolar capillaries. This adds desaturated venous blood into the pulmonary end-capillary blood, reducing its overall oxygen content. In normal subjects, thebesian and bronchial venous blood flows contribute to the small $(A - a)D_{O_2}$ seen in subjects with healthy lungs.

EFFECTS OF OXYGEN THERAPY IN LUNGS WITH VENTILATION–PERFUSION INEQUALITY AND SHUNT

When the gas exchange efficiency of the lung is reduced by shunt or ventilation–perfusion inequality, the arterial P_{O_2} decreases relative to the ideal alveolar P_{O_2}. When this occurs, supplemen-

Figure 7–9. The effects of ventilation with 100% oxygen in a lung with 35% shunt but no other V̇A/Q̇ inequality. *A.* During room air ventilation, blood exiting the nonventilated alveoli (1.75 liters/min with 59% oxygen saturation) mixes with blood exiting from the ideal alveoli (3.25 liters/min at 98% oxygen saturation) to produce arterial blood (5 liters/min at 84.5% oxygen saturation, Pao₂ = 50 torr). *B.* During ventilation with 100% oxygen, blood exiting from nonventilated alveoli (1.75 liters/min at 70% oxygen saturation) mixes with blood from ideal alveoli (3.25 liters/min at 100% oxygen saturation) to form systemic arterial blood (5 liters/min at 89% oxygen saturation). Note that C̄vo₂ is higher during oxygen ventilation because the oxygen therapy has caused an increase in the arterial O₂ content, thereby increasing systemic oxygen delivery. Note that V̇o₂ remains the same in *A* and *B*.

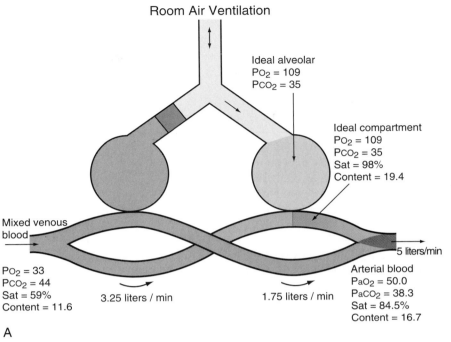

Room Air Ventilation

Ideal alveolar
$P_{O_2} = 109$
$P_{CO_2} = 35$

Ideal compartment
$P_{O_2} = 109$
$P_{CO_2} = 35$
Sat = 98%
Content = 19.4

Mixed venous blood

$P_{O_2} = 33$
$P_{CO_2} = 44$
Sat = 59%
Content = 11.6

3.25 liters / min

1.75 liters / min

5 liters/min

Arterial blood
$Pa_{O_2} = 50.0$
$Pa_{CO_2} = 38.3$
Sat = 84.5%
Content = 16.7

A

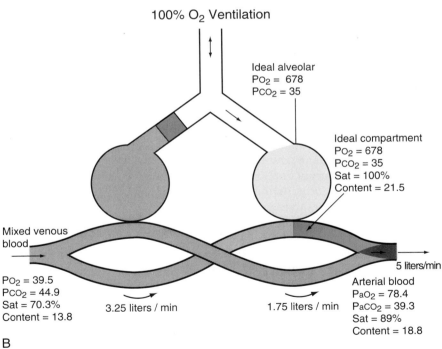

100% O₂ Ventilation

Ideal alveolar
$P_{O_2} = 678$
$P_{CO_2} = 35$

Ideal compartment
$P_{O_2} = 678$
$P_{CO_2} = 35$
Sat = 100%
Content = 21.5

Mixed venous blood

$P_{O_2} = 39.5$
$P_{CO_2} = 44.9$
Sat = 70.3%
Content = 13.8

3.25 liters / min

1.75 liters / min

5 liters/min

Arterial blood
$Pa_{O_2} = 78.4$
$Pa_{CO_2} = 39.3$
Sat = 89%
Content = 18.8

B

tary oxygen is sometimes used to increase the inspired, and thus the ideal alveolar P_{O_2}. This can increase the arterial P_{O_2}, although the magnitude of this increase depends in part on the cause of the gas exchange problem.

Oxygen Therapy in Pulmonary Shunting

Figure 7–9 compares the effects of ventilation with room air versus 100% oxygen in a lung with a 35% shunt. During room air ventilation (Figure 7–9A), blood exiting from the nonventilated alveoli has the same composition as mixed venous blood ($P\bar{v}_{O_2} = 33$ torr, $C\bar{v}_{O_2} = 11.6$ ml/dl). Blood exiting from the ideal alveoli is 98% saturated ($Cc'_{O_2} = 19.4$ ml/dl) and has the same P_{O_2} as that in the ideal alveolar gas ($P_{AO_2} = 109$ torr). The shunt blood flow (1.75 liters/min) mixes with blood flow from the ideal compartment (3.25 liters/min) to form arterial blood, whose oxygen content reflects a flow-weighted average of the two ($Ca_{O_2} = 16.7$ ml/dl). In this case, the average arterial oxygen content is associated with an arterial oxygen saturation of 85%, which corresponds to an arterial P_{O_2} of 50 torr. When the same lung is ventilated with 100% oxygen (Figure 7–9B), the alveolar P_{O_2} increases to 678 torr in the ventilated alveoli. Accordingly, the blood P_{O_2} exiting the ideal alveoli increases to the same level, and the oxygen content increases to 21.5 ml/dl. When this blood mixes with desaturated blood exiting from the nonventilated alveoli, the resulting arterial oxygen content now becomes 18.8 ml/dl. Since the cardiac output and oxygen uptake by the body ($\dot{V}_{O_2}$) remain constant, the mixed venous oxygen content will now increase slightly, because the arterial oxygen content has increased while the arteriovenous oxygen content difference has not changed. Hence, the mixed venous $P\bar{v}_{O_2}$ and oxygen content increase slightly. The final result is a greater arterial P_{O_2} (78 torr), a slightly greater mixed venous P_{O_2}, and the same 35% shunt. Although the arterial hypoxemia is improved, there is still a large $(A - a)D_{O_2}$ (600 torr).

In this example (see Figure 7–9), ventilation with supplemental oxygen produced a small but significant effect on the arterial P_{O_2}. Part of the reason for this relatively small improvement is that the blood leaving the ideal alveoli was nearly fully saturated with oxygen during room air ventilation. Therefore, pure oxygen did not substantially in-

crease the ideal end-capillary blood oxygen saturation. Most of the increase in ideal end-capillary oxygen content was caused by the additional dissolved oxygen, which results from the high ideal alveolar P_{O_2}. Obviously, ventilation with oxygen did not directly affect the oxygen content of blood from the nonventilated alveoli. However, ventilation with pure oxygen did increase the $P\bar{v}_{O_2}$ and oxygen content, because it increased systemic oxygen transport. In summary, when shunting is the primary cause of the arterial hypoxemia, supplemental oxygen has a relatively small effect on the arterial P_{O_2}. However, in patients with acute hypoxemic respiratory failure, this improvement can often mean the difference between an inadequate and a satisfactory level of arterial oxygenation.

Oxygen Therapy During Ventilation–Perfusion Inequality

Figure 7–10 shows the effect of supplemental oxygen therapy in a lung with ventilation–perfusion inequality but without shunt. In this lung, three populations of alveoli exist having $\dot{V}_A/\dot{Q}$ ratios of 0.05, 1.0, and 20. First consider the case during ventilation with room air. Because the $\dot{V}_A/\dot{Q}$ ratios among the compartments differ, the alveolar P_{O_2} values—and corresponding end-capillary P_{O_2} levels—also will differ. For example, in the $\dot{V}_A/\dot{Q} = 0.05$ compartment the alveolar P_{O_2} is 40 torr and end-capillary blood leaving these alveoli will be only 70% saturated (Figure 7–10A). Blood leaving the $\dot{V}_A/\dot{Q} = 1$ compartment will have a $P_{O_2} = 101$ torr and will be 97% saturated. Blood leaving the $\dot{V}_A/\dot{Q} = 20$ compartment will have a $P_{O_2} = 144$ and will be 99.4% saturated. If the blood flow is partitioned as shown, systemic arterial blood will be 91.5% saturated and will have a $Pa_{O_2} = 64.6$ torr. The ideal alveolar P_{O_2} for this lung would be 100 torr, according to the ideal alveolar oxygen equation. Note that arterial blood is incompletely saturated because desaturated blood from the $\dot{V}_A/\dot{Q} = 0.05$ alveoli has mixed with blood from the other two compartments. The $(A - a)D_{O_2}$ of 35 torr is a consequence of this $\dot{V}_A/\dot{Q}$ heterogeneity.

If this lung is ventilated with oxygen, the situation will change to that shown in Figure 7–10B. As before, the three populations of alveoli will have different alveolar P_{O_2} values by virtue of their different $\dot{V}_A/\dot{Q}$ ratios. However, since all alveoli re-

Figure 7–10. The effects of ventilation with 100% oxygen in a lung with ventilation–perfusion inequality, but no shunt. *A.* During room air ventilation, blood exiting from poorly ventilated alveoli (1.0 liter/min with 70% oxygen saturation) mixes with blood exiting from normally ventilated and perfused alveoli (3.95 liters/min at 97% oxygen saturation) and from excessively ventilated alveoli (0.05 liter/min at 99.4% saturation) to produce arterial blood (5 liters/min at 91.5% oxygen saturation, $Pa_{O_2} = 64.6$ torr). *B.* During ventilation with 100% oxygen, the alveolar P_{O_2} rises in all ventilated alveoli, even if they receive only a small amount of ventilation. Blood exiting from poorly ventilated alveoli (1.0 liter/min at $P_{O_2} = 661$ torr; oxygen saturation = 100%) mixes with blood from normally ventilated and perfused alveoli (3.95 liters/min at $P_{O_2} = 672$ torr; oxygen saturation = 100%) and from excessively ventilated alveoli (0.05 liter/min at $P_{O_2} = 702$ torr, oxygen saturation = 100%), yielding fully saturated mixed arterial blood ($Pa_{O_2} = 670$ torr). Thus, supplemental oxygen effectively reverses the arterial hypoxemia due to $\dot{V}_A/\dot{Q}$ inequality. Note that $\dot{V}_{O_2}$ remains the same in *A* and *B*.

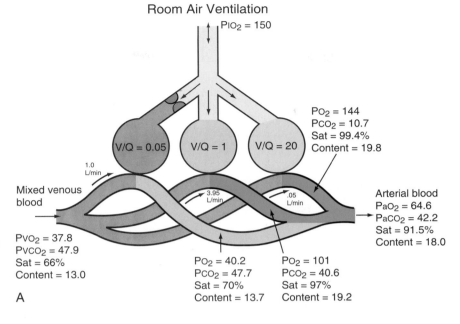

Room Air Ventilation

$PI_{O_2} = 150$

V/Q = 0.05   V/Q = 1   V/Q = 20

$P_{O_2} = 144$
$P_{CO_2} = 10.7$
Sat = 99.4%
Content = 19.8

1.0 L/min

Mixed venous blood

3.95 L/min   .05 L/min

Arterial blood
$Pa_{O_2} = 64.6$
$Pa_{CO_2} = 42.2$
Sat = 91.5%
Content = 18.0

$Pv_{O_2} = 37.8$
$Pv_{CO_2} = 47.9$
Sat = 66%
Content = 13.0

$P_{O_2} = 40.2$
$P_{CO_2} = 47.7$
Sat = 70%
Content = 13.7

$P_{O_2} = 101$
$P_{CO_2} = 40.6$
Sat = 97%
Content = 19.2

A

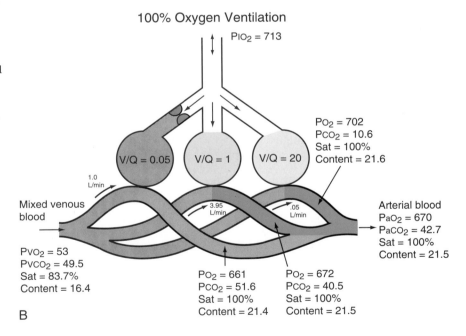

100% Oxygen Ventilation

$PI_{O_2} = 713$

V/Q = 0.05   V/Q = 1   V/Q = 20

$P_{O_2} = 702$
$P_{CO_2} = 10.6$
Sat = 100%
Content = 21.6

1.0 L/min

Mixed venous blood

3.95 L/min   .05 L/min

Arterial blood
$Pa_{O_2} = 670$
$Pa_{CO_2} = 42.7$
Sat = 100%
Content = 21.5

$Pv_{O_2} = 53$
$Pv_{CO_2} = 49.5$
Sat = 83.7%
Content = 16.4

$P_{O_2} = 661$
$P_{CO_2} = 51.6$
Sat = 100%
Content = 21.4

$P_{O_2} = 672$
$P_{CO_2} = 40.5$
Sat = 100%
Content = 21.5

B

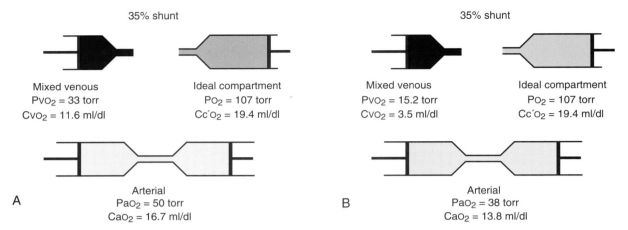

35% shunt

Mixed venous
$P\bar{v}_{O_2}$ = 33 torr
$C\bar{v}_{O_2}$ = 11.6 ml/dl

Ideal compartment
P_{O_2} = 107 torr
Cc'_{O_2} = 19.4 ml/dl

A

Arterial
Pa_{O_2} = 50 torr
Ca_{O_2} = 16.7 ml/dl

35% shunt

Mixed venous
$P\bar{v}_{O_2}$ = 15.2 torr
$C\bar{v}_{O_2}$ = 3.5 ml/dl

Ideal compartment
P_{O_2} = 107 torr
Cc'_{O_2} = 19.4 ml/dl

B

Arterial
Pa_{O_2} = 38 torr
Ca_{O_2} = 13.8 ml/dl

Figure 7–11. The effects of change in mixed venous blood oxygen content on the arterial P_{O_2} and content in a lung with 35% shunt. *A.* A 35% shunt with a cardiac output of 5 L/min. *B.* A 35% shunt with a cardiac output of 2.5 L/min. (See text for further explanation.)

ceive at least some ventilation, the alveolar P_{O_2} can be increased even in alveoli with very low $\dot{V}_A/\dot{Q}$ ratios. At this F_{IO_2}, the alveolar P_{O_2} in poorly ventilated alveoli can be increased enough to fully saturate end-capillary blood. As a result, mixed arterial blood no longer reflects the contribution of desaturated blood from poorly ventilated regions, and the arterial P_{O_2} increases to 670 torr. The $(A-a)D_{O_2}$ has decreased to less than 1 torr, although the lung has not changed its overall efficiency of gas exchange. Thus, it can be said that oxygen is an effective means of increasing the arterial P_{O_2} in lungs with ventilation–perfusion inequality.

EFFECTS OF MIXED VENOUS OXYGEN CONTENT

Depending on its $\dot{V}_A/\dot{Q}$ ratio, the P_{O_2} in a single alveolus can be as small as mixed venous P_{O_2} (when $\dot{V}_A/\dot{Q} = 0$) or as great as the inspired P_{O_2} (when $\dot{V}_A/\dot{Q} = \infty$).When shunting is present in the lungs, desaturated (mixed venous) blood exiting from nonventilated (shunt) alveoli admixes with well-oxygenated blood coming from the normally ventilated alveoli. Hence, the lower the oxygen content of mixed venous blood, the lower the content of systemic arterial blood will be for a given amount of

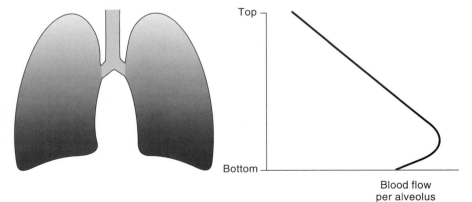

Figure 7–12. Topographical distribution of blood flow from the apex to the base of a vertical lung. Blood flow per alveolus increases from the top to the bottom of the lung due to the effects of gravity on the pulmonary circulation (see Chapter 4).

Top

Bottom

Blood flow per alveolus

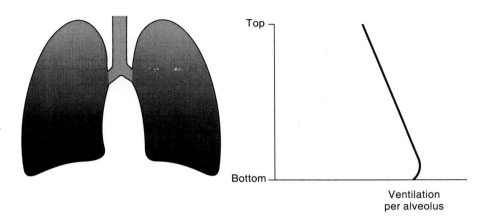

Figure 7–13. Ventilation per alveolus from the apex to the base of a vertical lung. Higher transpulmonary pressures near the top of the lung cause the alveoli near the apex to have larger volume at functional residual capacity, but they change their volume less during inspiration because they operate higher on their pressure–volume relationships (see Chapter 1). Hence, their ventilation per unit volume (effective alveolar ventilation) is less than for alveoli at the bottom of the lung because of effects of gravity.

shunt. Factors that increase mixed venous oxygen content (e.g., increases in cardiac output) will increase the arterial oxygen content and Po_2, whereas factors that decrease the oxygen content in mixed venous blood (e.g., reduced cardiac output or increased $\dot{V}o_2$) will reduce the arterial blood content, for a given percent shunt. Figure 7–11 shows the effect of mixed venous oxygenation on the arterial oxygenation in a lung with a 35% shunt. In Figure 7–11A, blood exiting from nonventilated alveoli has a Po_2 of 33 torr (35% saturation), while blood from the ideal alveoli has a Po_2 of 107 torr (98% saturation). Mixed arterial blood has an oxygen saturation of 86%, corresponding to an arterial Po_2 of 50 torr. In the same lung, if the cardiac output is decreased by 50%, mixed venous oxygen saturation decreases to 18% ($P\overline{v}o_2 = 15.2$ torr), then the mixed arterial oxygen saturation will decrease to 70.3% ($Pao_2 = 38$ torr) even though the shunt stays at 35%. Thus, factors that increase or decrease mixed venous oxygen content will tend to increase or decrease the arterial oxygen saturation and Po_2 for a given amount of shunt. This is also true when the hypoxemia is due to $\dot{V}A/\dot{Q}$ inequality without shunt.

VENTILATION–PERFUSION INEQUALITY IN NORMAL LUNGS

An ideal lung is one where the $(A-a)Do_2$ is zero. As shown earlier, this occurs when all of the alveoli in the lung operate at the same $\dot{V}A/\dot{Q}$ ratio. However,

even healthy lungs show a small difference between ideal alveolar Po_2 and arterial Po_2, because of differences in $\dot{V}A/\dot{Q}$ ratios that exist among alveoli. This small amount of $\dot{V}A/\dot{Q}$ heterogeneity occurs

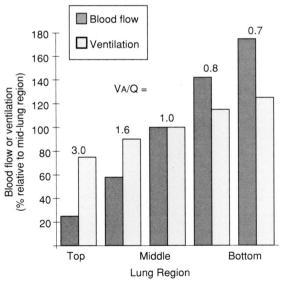

Figure 7–14. Relative ventilation, blood flow, and $\dot{V}A/\dot{Q}$ ratio from the base to the apex of a vertical lung. Alveoli at the bottom of the lung receive more blood flow than ventilation and thus have $\dot{V}A/\dot{Q}$ ratios of less than 1.0. Alveoli near the top of the lung normally receive somewhat less ventilation than at the base, but they receive much less blood flow. Hence, alveoli near the top have $\dot{V}A/\dot{Q}$ ratios in the range of 1 to 10. Under some circumstances (e.g., hemorrhage), alveoli at the apex may receive some ventilation but no blood flow at all, giving rise to alveoli with $\dot{V}A/\dot{Q} = \infty$.

because of the effects of gravity on the distribution of blood flow and ventilation in the lung.

Figure 7–12 shows the distribution of blood flow from the base to the apex of a vertical lung (see Chapter 4). Blood flow per alveolus increases toward the base of the vertical lung. This results from the changes in perfusing pressures and, in part, from the recruitment and distention of vessels closer to the base of the lung. These differences in alveolar blood flow result from the effects of gravity. Gravity also influences the distribution of alveolar ventilation in a vertical lung, as detailed in Chapter 1. Figure 7–13 shows that the ventilation per alveolus is greater near the base of a vertical lung than at the apex.

Although both the ventilation and blood flow per alveolus decrease from the top to the bottom of the lung, the change in blood flow is relatively more marked than the change in ventilation. Therefore, the ratio of ventilation to blood flow varies from the top to the bottom of the lung. Figure 7–14 shows the effect of these regional differences in ventilation and blood flow on the local $\dot{V}A/\dot{Q}$ ratio from the bottom to the top of a vertical lung. The small dispersion of $\dot{V}A/\dot{Q}$ that results from the effects of gravity is largely responsible for the small (A − a)Do_2 (2 to 4 torr) typically found in normal subjects with healthy lungs.

Since the lung is longer than it is wide, the regional differences in the $\dot{V}A/\dot{Q}$ ratio are most evident in a subject who is standing. When the same subject lies down, gradients in blood flow and ventilation still occur between anterior and posterior levels, but the magnitude of the differences in regional ventilation and blood flow is smaller because the vertical distances are smaller. Accordingly, lung gas exchange becomes more homogeneous in a recumbent subject because there is less variation in the $\dot{V}A/\dot{Q}$ among regions in the lung.

Chapter 8

Control of Ventilation

The rate, depth, and pattern of breathing are determined by the coordinated contraction of the muscles of the diaphragm, chest wall, abdomen, and surrounding structures. The coordinated control of the respiratory muscles for breathing and speech production is a complex process that requires the input and processing of large amounts of information by the respiratory control center in the brain stem. The physiological regulation of the rate, depth, and pattern of breathing reflects the integration of information originating in (1) multiple higher regions of the central nervous system; (2) chemosensitive receptors located within the central nervous system and also in the aortic arch and carotid arteries; (3) neural receptors located in the lung itself; (4) neural mechanoreceptors located in skin, pharynx, larynx, and the airways; and (5) other receptors located within the thoracic cavity. The term *control of ventilation* refers to the generation and regulation of periodic breathing by the respiratory center in the brain stem and its modification by the input of information from higher brain centers and systemic receptors. This chapter begins with an overview of the major systems known to contribute to the control of ventilation. Next, the major individual components of the system are examined in greater detail. Finally, examples of the integrated ventilatory responses to specific interventions are considered and known defects in the control of ventilation are examined.

OVERVIEW OF VENTILATORY CONTROL

A schematic overview of the ventilatory control system is presented in Figure 8–1. This represents a functional, rather than an anatomical, description of the neural centers that participate in ventilatory

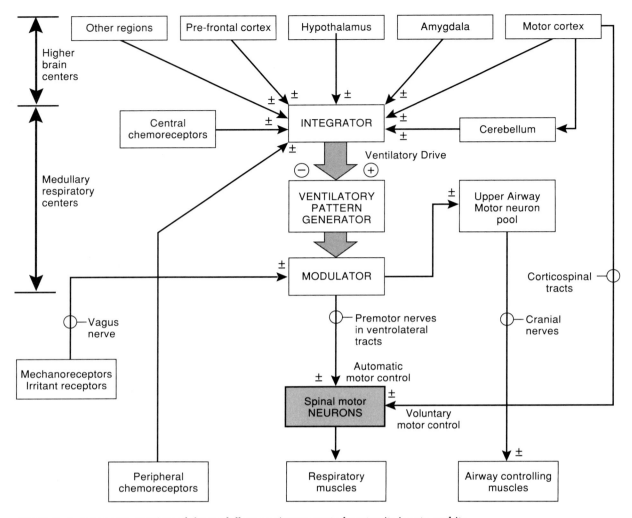

Figure 8-1. Schematic overview of the medullary respiratory control center, its inputs, and its output to the motor neurons controlling the muscles of respiration. Note that voluntary control of the respiratory muscles competes with automatic ventilatory control at the level of the respiratory muscle motor neurons. See text for further explanation.

control. The central component of this system resides in the medulla oblongata of the brain stem and is termed the *respiratory control center*. This control center is a collection of several anatomically distinct groups of nerve cells (termed *nuclei*) that act to generate and modify the basic rhythmic ventilatory pattern. The *ventilatory pattern generator* is the central site where the rhythmic pattern of ventilation is created in the medulla. The rate and amplitude of this ventilatory pattern is controlled by the output

of an *integrator*, which processes inputs from higher brain centers and chemoreceptors.

The integrator effectively determines the appropriate *ventilatory drive* (stimulation) for the pattern generator based on the requirements for ventilation arising from higher brain centers. Activity in cerebral cortex, hypothalamus, amygdala, the limbic system, and cerebellum can modify ventilatory drive in response to visual, emotional, painful, or voluntary motor stimuli. For example, severe visceral pain stimulates ventilation; emotional upset may elicit involuntary hyperventilation, and sudden visual stimuli may elicit transient inspiration. Indeed, the very act of thinking about one's breathing can alter the respiratory pattern. Postural adjustments, voluntary body movement, and speech will modify the breathing pattern and pattern formation as part of the coordination of movement and breathing. Neural inputs from the cerebellum influence the ventilatory drive in the coordination of breathing with postural adjustments or other body movements. The reticular activating system can influence the ventilatory drive during sleep. For example, during slow-wave sleep the pattern of ventilation is relatively uniform, whereas during rapid eye movement sleep, it is more variable.

Specialized chemoreceptive cells (peripheral chemoreceptors) located in the aortic arch (aortic bodies) and at the bifurcation of the internal and external carotid arteries in the neck (carotid bodies) sense the Po_2, Pco_2, and pH of arterial blood. This feedback information is transmitted back to the drive integration nuclei in the medulla through cranial nerves. Information from the aortic bodies travels to the central nervous system in the vagus nerve. Information from the carotid bodies travels in the carotid sinus nerve, which is a branch of the glossopharyngeal nerve. Chemoreceptors located just below the ventrolateral surface of the medulla (central chemoreceptors) detect changes in the Pco_2/pH of brain stem interstitial fluid. This information is also integrated into the determination of ventilatory drive. For example, in states in which the arterial Pco_2 is abnormally high, increased activity from central and peripheral chemoreceptors causes the integrated ventilatory drive to increase. This stimulates the pattern generator to produce an increased tidal volume and frequency of ventilation.

Other regions modulate the optimal pattern generated by the respiratory pattern generator. For example, mechanoreceptors and irritant receptors in the airways can modify the ventilatory pattern in accord with the degree of lung inflation or the presence of an irritating substance in the airways. The modulated output of the pattern generator represents the collective output of the respiratory control center to the motor neurons that control the muscles of inspiration and expiration.

Ultimately, minute ventilation is effected by the contraction of the striated muscles of respiration, which are under the control of their respective motor neurons. The motor neurons controlling respiratory muscles of the chest wall are located in the anterior horn of the spinal column. Intercostal muscles and the accessory muscles of respiration are controlled by motor neurons located in the thoracic region of the spinal column. Diaphragmatic motor neurons are situated in the cervical region of the spine and control the diaphragm bilaterally through the phrenic nerves.

Voluntary motor control of the diaphragm, intercostals, and other muscles of ventilation originates in the motor cortex. This information passes directly to the motor neurons in the spine through the corticospinal tracts, thus bypassing the medullary respiratory control center. The respiratory muscle motor neurons act as the final site of integration of voluntary (corticospinal tract) and automatic (ventrolateral tracts) control of ventilation. Voluntary control of these muscles competes with automatic influences at the level of the spinal motor neuron. The concept of competing voluntary and automatic control of the respiratory muscles is demonstrated clearly if a subject attempts a breath-holding maneuver. Voluntary control can dominate the spinal motor neurons at first, but the influence of automatic ventilatory control eventually overpowers the voluntary effort and limits how long the breath can be held.

The motor neurons innervating muscles in the upper airways (airway controlling muscles) are situated within the medulla near the respiratory control center. These motor neurons innervate muscles in the upper airways and bronchi through cranial nerves. Activation of these muscles occurs a few tenths of a second before the major muscles of inspiration are activated, causing dilation of the pharynx and large airways at the initiation of inspiration.

VENTILATORY RESPONSES TO CARBON DIOXIDE AND OXYGEN

Figure 8-2 shows the ventilatory response to changes in arterial Po_2 at a normal level of arterial Pco_2. To generate this response, ventilation is measured in a subject breathing a low inspired oxygen

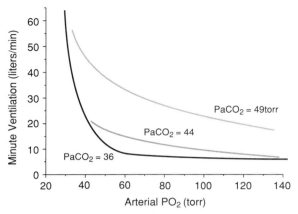

Figure 8–2. The ventilatory response to reduced arterial oxygen tension. This response is mediated exclusively by the peripheral chemoreceptors. Simultaneous increases in arterial $Paco_2$ amplify the ventilatory response to hypoxia. The small numbers adjacent to each curve refer to the constant $Paco_2$ that was maintained as alveolar Po_2 was progressively reduced. At a normal $Paco_2$ (36 torr), reduced oxygen tension does not stimulate ventilation until arterial or Pao_2 is less than 60 torr.

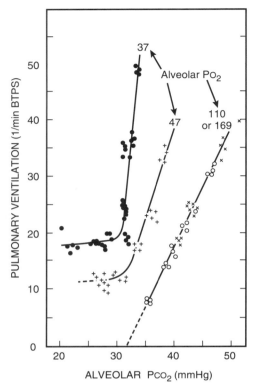

Figure 8–3. The ventilatory response to carbon dioxide. This response is mediated by the central and peripheral chemoreceptors. Simultaneous decreases in arterial Po_2 amplify the ventilatory response to increased Pco_2. The small numbers adjacent to each curve refer to the constant Po_2 that was maintained as alveolar Pco_2 was progressively increased. (Redrawn from Nielsen M, Smith H: Studies on the regulation of respiration in acute hypoxia. Acta Physiol Scand 24:293, 1951.)

gas mixture to which carbon dioxide has been added to maintain a normal arterial Pco_2. The decrease in arterial Po_2 is detected by the peripheral chemoreceptors, which increase their rate of firing in response to the reduced Po_2. Note that *hypoxemia* (decreased arterial Po_2) does not begin to stimulate ventilation until the arterial Po_2 falls below about 60 torr. Below this tension, further reduction in arterial Po_2 elicits a marked stimulation in minute ventilation. However, if arterial Pco_2 is maintained at an increased level as Po_2 is reduced, the ventilatory stimulation is markedly increased.

The regulation of carbon dioxide tension and blood pH is essential for the normal function of many enzymes and other cell proteins of the body. The respiratory control system regulates minute ventilation in an attempt to control arterial Pco_2 (and thus pH) within the normal range. Changes in arterial Pco_2 are detected by both the central and peripheral chemoreceptors, which transmit this information to the medullary respiratory centers. This information is integrated by the central nervous system in its synthesis of ventilatory drive. Figure 8–3 shows the change in ventilation that occurs in response to induced changes in the level of arterial Pco_2. To generate this response, the inspired oxygen and carbon dioxide concentrations are adjusted to produce an increase in arterial Pco_2 while main-

taining a constant arterial Po_2. At high levels of arterial Po_2, ventilation increases linearly with increases in Pco_2. The slope of this response reflects the amount that ventilation increases for a given change in Pco_2 and is termed the *ventilatory response to carbon dioxide*. Note that when low arterial Po_2 is combined with increases in Pco_2, the ventilatory response to carbon dioxide is augmented significantly. Likewise, when Pco_2 is increased, the ventilatory response to oxygen is augmented. This amplifying effect occurs because separate mechanisms are responsible for sensing Pco_2 and Po_2 in the peripheral chemoreceptors. Hence, the presence of both hypercapnia and hypoxemia can have an additive effect on chemoreceptor output and the resulting ventilatory stimulation.

Anesthetic agents, narcotics, barbiturates, and other depressants of the central nervous system suppress the ventilatory responses to oxygen and carbon dioxide. Figure 8–4 shows this effect as a reduction in the ventilatory drive for carbon dioxide compared with a normal subject. In this state, an inadequate stimulus is generated to drive the motor neurons innervating the muscles of respiration. As a consequence, ventilation is inadequate to maintain an appropriate amount of carbon dioxide excretion, and arterial hypercapnia results.

Mechanical factors interfering with airflow in the lung can also reduce the ventilatory response to oxygen and carbon dioxide. In patients with partial airflow obstruction or increased work of breathing, the ventilatory response to increased carbon dioxide may be blunted, even though the medullary respi-

ratory control centers may be normal. In this situation, the stimulus to the respiratory motor neurons is normal but the amount of ventilation generated is less because of the mechanical restriction to ventilation.

ORGANIZATION OF THE MEDULLARY RESPIRATORY CONTROL CENTER

The rhythmic respiratory pattern originates in the medulla oblongata of the brain stem. Studies in animals using focal cell destruction (*ablation*) or surgical cross-cutting of the brain stem (*sectioning*) have found that sectioning the spinal column at the caudal (toward the tail) end of the medulla ablated all periodic breathing. However, if the spinal column is sectioned instead at the junction of the medulla and pons, periodic breathing is retained (although the pattern of breathing is altered). From this, it has been concluded that the inherent rhythmicity of breathing originates in the medulla. Recent electrophysiological studies have shown that groups of neurons in several different medullary nuclei increase their frequency of action potentials (rate of firing) during inspiration, whereas other groups of cells increase their rate of firing during expiration. Unlike the heart, no single group of pacemaker cells in the medulla appears responsible for the basic rhythmic pattern of ventilation. Rather, the inspiratory-expiratory pattern is generated by groups of interconnected nerves, termed *neural networks*, that act as oscillating circuits. Within these networks, the frequency of firing increases in various cells at different points during inspiration, while other groups of cells become active at various points during expiration. Duplicate sets of these neural oscillator networks must exist in the medulla, since focal injury to a single location fails to halt the generation of a normal respiratory rhythm.

Most of the cells involved in respiratory pattern generation are located within two distinct nuclei within the medulla. A *dorsal respiratory group* is composed of cells in the *nucleus tractus solitarius* located in the dorsomedial region of the medulla. Cells in the dorsal respiratory group appear active primarily during inspiration. A *ventral respiratory group* is located in the ventrolateral region of the medulla and is composed of three separate nuclei. The rostral *nucleus retrofacialis* and the caudal *nu-*

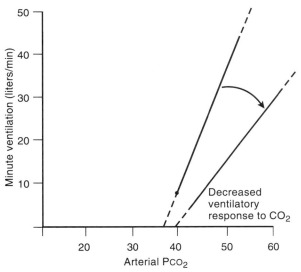

Figure 8–4. Decreased ventilatory response to carbon dioxide caused by central nervous system depressants or airflow obstruction. Drugs such as barbiturates and narcotics depress central nervous system activity and can reduce the ventilatory response to increased P_{CO_2}. Ventilation is reduced as a function of increased P_{CO_2} because the stimulus driving the respiratory motor neurons is inadequate to maintain normal ventilation. In the *absence* of respiratory depressants, subjects with increased work of breathing (resulting from airflow obstruction, for example) can show a similar reduction in the ventilatory response to carbon dioxide. However, in these subjects the signal to the motor neurons is normal but the ventilation achieved is reduced.

cleus retroambiguus appear active during expiration, whereas the middle *nucleus para-ambiguus* is most active during inspiration. Active discharge by cells in these nuclei appears to excite activity in some cells and to inhibit activity in others.

During the respiratory cycle, the medullary respiratory centers transmit a characteristic pattern of activity to the motor neurons supplying the muscles of inspiration. As shown in Figure 8–5, this pattern can be divided into one inspiratory and two expiratory phases. The *inspiratory phase* begins with an abrupt increase in discharge frequency, followed by a steady ramplike increase in firing rate through the remainder of inspiration. During automatic breathing, this leads to the progressive contraction of the inspiratory muscles. The end of inspiration is signaled by an *off-switch* event, which abruptly decreases the firing rate. At the start of expiration, there is a paradoxical increase in the activity to inspiratory motor neurons (*expiratory phase I*). This activity tends to slow down or "brake" the early phase of expiration by augmenting inspiratory muscle tone. Inspiratory activity is completely absent during the latter phase of expiration (*expiratory phase II*). When ventilation is increased as in exercise, active stimulation of the expiratory muscles occurs only during the second expiratory phase. Neural recordings have demonstrated that approximately six different cell types in the dorsal and ventral regulatory groups contribute to the different parts of the composite inspiratory premotor activity shown in Figure 8–5. This is significant, because stimulation of a single cell type can markedly influence the ventilatory pattern. For example, the Hering-Breuer reflex is an inspiratory-inhibitory reflex that arises from afferent stretch receptors located in the smooth muscle of the airways. Progressive increases in lung inflation tend to stretch these receptors and promote an earlier expiration by exciting neurons associated with the off-switch phase of inspiratory muscle control.

PERIPHERAL CHEMORECEPTORS

The carotid and aortic bodies are highly specialized chemical receptors that continuously sense the Po_2, Pco_2 and pH of arterial blood and transmit related afferent information back to the medullary respiratory centers. Peripheral chemoreceptors are small,

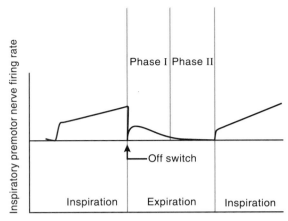

Figure 8–5. Neural signal driving the inspiratory motor neurons. This signal driving the inspiratory muscles can be divided into one *inspiratory* and two *expiratory* phases. This pattern of neural activity represents the composite of contributions from several different cell types in the medullary respiratory control center. See text for further explanation.

highly vascular structures that are highly responsive to arterial Po_2 and Pco_2 and are also responsive to arterial pH. Because the central chemoreceptors are not sensitive to Po_2, the peripheral chemoreceptors provide the only sensitivity to low arterial Po_2. Normally, the peripheral chemoreceptors are responsible for about 40% of the ventilatory response to carbon dioxide; the balance is provided by the central chemoreceptors (see later).

Despite decades of study, the precise mechanisms underlying the detection of pH, Pco_2, and Po_2 are still not fully understood. Figure 8–6 illustrates the primary structures present in the carotid body. Type I (*glomus*) cells are rich in mitochondria and endoplasmic reticulum and contain several different types of cytoplasmic granules (*synaptic vesicles*). The synaptic vesicles contain different neurotransmitters, including dopamine, acetylcholine, norepinephrine, and neuropeptides. Type I cells are the primary site for transducing the local pH, Pco_2, and Po_2. Afferent nerve terminals synapse with the type I cells and transmit information back to the brain stem through the carotid sinus nerve. Vascular channels lined with endothelium convey blood flow at high rates in close proximity to type I cells, allowing the receptors to sense the gas tensions and pH of arterial blood. These structures are enveloped

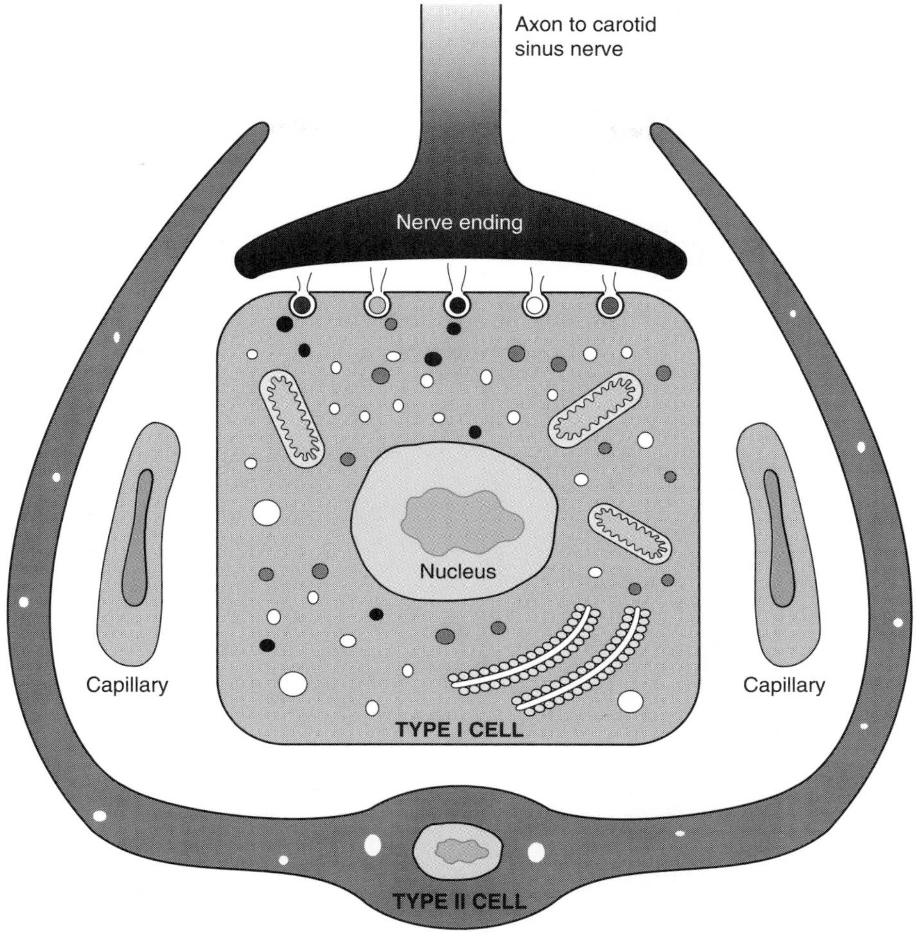

Figure 8-6. Structure of the carotid bodies. The carotid bodies are small, highly vascular tissues composed of several different cell types. Type I (glomus) cells are metabolically active and contain large numbers of synaptic vesicles containing neurotransmitters. Increased Pco_2, decreased pH, or decreased Po_2 in arterial blood causes the release of multiple neurotransmitters from the glomus cells that act on adjacent nerve terminals. Activity generated in these nerve terminals is transmitted to the medullary respiratory control center through the carotid sinus nerve. Type II cells envelop these structures.

by long cytoplasmic extensions from type II cells, which generally resemble neural *Schwann cells.*

Detection of low arterial Po_2 by the peripheral chemoreceptors has been linked to a decrease in cellular adenosine triphosphate (ATP) levels. Cyanide, a metabolic inhibitor of mitochondrial electron transport, is a potent stimulant of carotid sinus nerve activity and ventilation because it rapidly reduces the ATP concentration in type I cells. Low arterial Po_2 also causes a decrease in the ATP concentration in type I cells. This leads to a depolarization of the cell and the subsequent release of one or more neurotransmitters that act on the afferent nerve terminals. Detection of Pco_2 and pH occurs by inducing changes in the intracellular pH of type I cells, which causes release of other neurotransmit-

ters. The same type I cells are responsive to low Po_2, decreased pH, and increased arterial Pco_2. [Hence, the activity in an afferent chemoreceptor nerve fiber will increase further if low arterial Po_2 is superimposed on a Pco_2 that was increased at the outset.]

CEREBROSPINAL FLUID AND THE CENTRAL CHEMORECEPTORS

The brain and spinal cord are bathed by a protein-free fluid that is continuously secreted by the *choroid plexus* and reabsorbed at the *arachnoid villi.* Termed *cerebrospinal fluid* (CSF), this liquid is an ultrafiltrate of plasma that is replaced by newly secreted CSF every few hours. Cerebrospinal fluid is in contact with extracellular fluid in the brain, and its composition therefore reflects the conditions surrounding the cells in the brain. Although formed from the blood, the ionic composition of CSF is not identical with that in plasma. A barrier with a low permeability to ions termed the *blood-brain barrier* separates blood and CSF. The blood–brain barrier is composed of endothelium, vascular smooth muscle, and the pial and arachnoid membranes. These membranes control the ionic composition of CSF by limiting the entrance of ions through specific membrane ion transporters (Figure 8–7). In addition, the ionic composition of CSF is regulated by the choroid plexus, which determines the composition of CSF as it is formed. Carbon dioxide diffuses rapidly across the blood–brain barrier, and the P_{CO_2} in the CSF parallels the arterial P_{CO_2} tension. Because the brain cells continuously release carbon dioxide as a product of metabolism, the P_{CO_2} of CSF is normally a few torr higher than arterial P_{CO_2}, and the pH is slightly more acidic than in plasma.

The *central chemoreceptors* are specialized groups

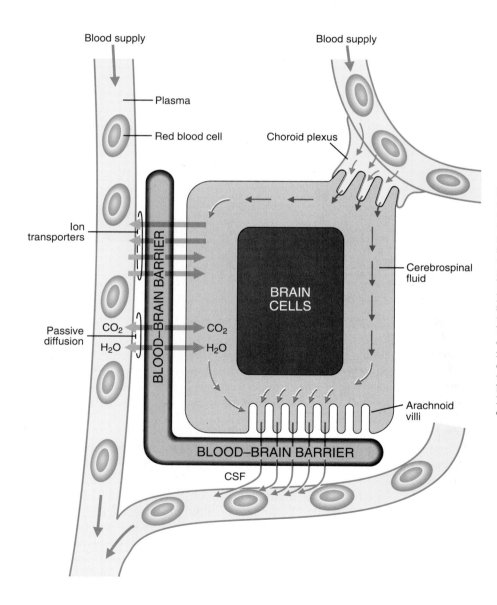

Figure 8–7. Control of cerebrospinal fluid (CSF) composition. CSF is secreted by the choroid plexus from plasma and bathes the central nervous system. Its composition reflects the extracellular environment for the brain cells. The blood–brain barrier has a low permeability to ions and separates blood from CSF. Ion transporters in the blood–brain barrier can alter the ionic composition of CSF, thereby regulating its pH. Carbon dioxide diffuses rapidly through the blood–brain barrier, so changes in arterial P_{CO_2} produce rapid parallel changes in the P_{CO_2} of the CSF.

of cells located within the ventrolateral surface of the medulla that are sensitive to the pH of the extracellular fluid around them. Since the extracellular fluid is in contact with CSF, changes in the pH of CSF can affect ventilation by acting on these chemoreceptive cells. The pH of CSF is related to the bicarbonate ion concentration $[HCO_3^-]$ and P_{CO_2} within CSF by the Henderson-Hasselbach equation:

$$pH = pK + \log \frac{[HCO_3^-]}{\alpha \cdot P_{CO_2}}$$

where α is a solubility coefficient of 0.03 mmol $\cdot$ liter^{-1} $\cdot$ torr^{-1} and pK is the negative log of the dissociation constant for carbonic acid. From this equation, it can be seen that increases in the P_{CO_2} will cause a decrease in the pH of the CSF at a given bicarbonate concentration. Likewise, increases in CSF bicarbonate concentration will increase pH in the CSF at any given P_{CO_2}. Increases in arterial P_{CO_2} cause the P_{CO_2} in the CSF to increase, producing a decrease in CSF pH. Conversely, decreases in arterial P_{CO_2} produce a rapid decrease in the P_{CO_2} in the CSF and cause an acute alkalosis in CSF.

EXAMPLE. Calculate the pH in blood if the plasma bicarbonate concentration is 24 mmol/liter, the P_{CO_2} is 40 torr, and the pK is 6.1

$$pH = 6.1 + \log (24/(40 \cdot 0.03))$$
$$pH = 6.1 + 1.3 = 7.4$$

What would the pH be if the P_{CO_2} remained at 40 torr but the bicarbonate concentration decreased to 18 mmol/liter?

$$pH = 6.1 + \log (18/(40 \cdot 0.03))$$
$$pH = 6.1 + 1.18 = 7.28 \qquad \blacksquare$$

To protect the brain under conditions in which the arterial P_{CO_2} is abnormally altered, the blood–brain barrier regulates the pH of CSF (normally about 7.33) by adjusting the ionic composition and bicarbonate concentration of CSF. However, changes in the CSF bicarbonate concentration occur slowly and take many hours to return the pH toward normal. Adjustments in ventilation may reflect differences in the information arising from central and peripheral chemoreceptors, as illustrated in the following example.

EXAMPLE. Consider the ventilatory changes that would occur in a group of healthy medical students during a weekend sojourn from Los Angeles (sea level, barometric pressure = 760 torr) up Mt. Whitney (altitude, 14,000 ft; barometric pressure, 460 torr). While breathing air at sea level

$$\text{Inspired } P_{O_2} (P_{IO_2}) = (760 - 47) \times 0.209$$
$$= 149 \text{ torr}$$

Assuming that ventilation is normal, arterial (and alveolar) P_{CO_2} will average about 40 torr, so the ideal alveolar P_{O_2} ($P_{AO_2} = P_{IO_2} - P_{ACO_2}/R$) will be approximately $149 - 40/0.8 = 99$ Torr. Assuming an average $(A - a)D_{O_2}$ of 5 torr, these students will have arterial P_{O_2} values of about 94 torr in Los Angeles. The students drive from Los Angeles to Loma Portal (altitude, 8,000 ft) on Saturday morning and hike up to the summit (barometric pressure = 460 torr), where they camp for the night. In camp

$$\text{Inspired } P_{O_2} = (460 - 47) \times 0.209 = 86 \text{ torr}$$

If the students' alveolar P_{CO_2} had remained at 40 torr, then the ideal alveolar P_{O_2} would have been $86 - 40/.8 = 36$ torr. However, the peripheral chemoreceptors should stimulate ventilation if the arterial P_{O_2} falls below approximately 60 torr, causing the alveolar (and arterial) P_{CO_2} to decrease. If arterial P_{CO_2} decreases to 20 torr, then ideal alveolar P_{O_2} would be $86 - 25/0.8 = 55$ torr, and arterial P_{O_2} would be a few torr less than this. Note that the decrease in arterial P_{CO_2} caused by the increased ventilation causes a decrease in the P_{CO_2} of the CSF and a corresponding increase in the pH of the CSF. This CSF alkalosis tends to attenuate the rate of discharge of central chemoreceptors and decreases their contribution to ventilatory drive. During the night, ion pumps in the blood–brain barrier cause a gradual reduction in the bicarbonate concentration in the CSF. This causes a decrease in the bicarbonate ion concentration in the CSF and a corresponding return of pH in the CSF toward normal. As this occurs, the inhibition of central chemoreceptor activity is removed and the corresponding increase in their firing further augments the minute ventilation. Likewise, the gradual excretion of bicarbonate ions from plasma by the kidney tends to return blood pH back toward normal. This augments peripheral chemoreceptor activity and ventilation by removing the inhibitory effect of a high arterial pH and low arterial P_{CO_2}. By Sunday morning, minute ventilation will have increased above the level of the previous evening at that altitude because of the increase in central and peripheral chemoreceptor firing as CSF and plasma pH return toward normal. Thus, the maximum increase in minute ventilation at a given altitude is not achieved until 18 to 36 hours because of the slow adjustments in the pH of CSF and blood.

Because classes resume on Monday, the students begin their descent to sea level on Sunday afternoon. They descend from the mountain quickly and then drive back to sea level. On return to low altitude, the inspired P_{O_2} returns to a normal value and the hypoxic stimulus to ventilation disappears. As arterial P_{O_2} increases toward normal levels, ventilation slows because the peripheral chemoreceptor rate of firing decreases. This causes the alveolar and arterial P_{CO_2} to increase toward the normal value of 40 torr. The increase in arterial P_{CO_2} is transmitted across the blood–brain barrier and causes the P_{CO_2} in the CSF to increase. This causes the pH in the CSF to decrease below normal levels, because the CSF bicarbonate concentration is low. [Recall that the bicarbonate concentration was previously reduced in an attempt to restore the pH in the CSF in the presence of low P_{CO_2}.] Consequently, ventilation is still augmented on return to sea level, because the low pH in the CSF continues to stimulate central chemoreceptors. Similarly, the pH in blood is decreased because the plasma bicarbonate concentration is decreased. [Recall that bicarbonate ions were previously excreted by the kidney to restore a normal blood pH in the presence of low P_{aCO_2}.] During the next 18 to 36 hours, bicarbonate ions are returned to the CSF from the blood and the kidney reabsorbs bicarbonate ions from glomerular filtrate. This restores a normal pH in the CSF and plasma and removes the residual stimulus to ventilation caused by low pH in central and peripheral chemo-

receptors. Hence, ventilation is not fully restored to normal values until 18 to 36 hours after return to low altitude.

SYSTEMIC RECEPTORS AND VENTILATORY REFLEXES

Several different types of sensory receptors in extrapulmonary airways contribute to the reflex control of ventilation by modulating ventilatory patterns. For example, stimulation of nasal or facial receptors with cold water initiates the *diving reflex.* This reflex elicits a cessation of ventilation *(apnea)* and bradycardia and is especially marked in newborns. *Irritant receptors* in the nose and upper airways are responsible for the reflex apnea elicited by inhalation of substances such as ammonia. Other receptors in the pharynx and upper airways mediate reflex changes in ventilation in response to swallowing, gagging, and aspiration.

Sensory nerve endings within the lungs and airways also contribute to the reflex modulation of ventilation. Fibers from these receptors travel to the medulla through the vagus nerve. *Slowly adapting receptors* maintain a constant rate of firing as a function of lung volume, while *rapidly adapting fibers* respond only as lung volume is changing (see Chapter 12). The former provide the respiratory control center with information related to the volume state of the lung, while the latter appear to be involved in augmented breaths (e.g., sighs). Slowly adapting receptors in airways provide the afferent limb of the Hering-Breuer inspiratory-inhibitory reflex. Increases in lung volume stimulate these receptors and elicit a cessation of inspiration by stimulating off-switch neurons in the medulla. The Hering-Breuer reflex is most effective when ventilatory rate and tidal volume are increased but is relatively inactive during quiet breathing.

Specialized receptors in the airways mediate the ventilatory responses elicited by inhalation of irritating substances such as chemicals, noxious gases, and even cold air. These receptors transmit information through unmyelinated C-fibers in the vagus nerve. Similar receptors in the lung parenchyma termed *juxta-alveolar* or *J receptors* are sensitive to chemical or mechanical stimulation in the lung interstitium. These receptors may mediate the altered breathing patterns seen in interstitial lung edema or in states of lung inflammation.

Somatic receptors in the intercostal muscles, rib joints, accessory muscles of respiration, and tendons can provide information on the length–tension control of the respiratory muscles. However, the role played by these receptors is more directly involved in postural and voluntary movement control than in the regulation of respiratory efforts per se. The diaphragm has fewer such receptors and is not directly involved in postural control.

CONTROL OF VENTILATION DURING EXERCISE

During exercise, the uptake of oxygen in working muscle increases because the metabolic rate increases. Carbon dioxide released during metabolism diffuses from the muscle into blood and is transported to the lung for elimination. At mild to moderate exercise intensity, alveolar ventilation increases in proportion to the increased carbon dioxide production, and arterial P_{CO_2} remains at normal levels. However, the mechanisms responsible for the increased ventilation during exercise are not understood fully. No single mediator or mechanism has been identified to explain why ventilation remains closely matched to the carbon dioxide production. Since arterial P_{O_2} and P_{CO_2} remain at normal levels, hypercapnic or hypoxic stimulation of chemoreceptors is not the mechanism. Mechanisms believed to contribute include neural inputs from the motor cortex to the medullary respiratory control center, afferents from muscle and joint mechanoreceptors, or unknown mediators released from working muscles. Whatever the mechanism, it operates as if it were able to adjust alveolar ventilation in proportion to the increased flux of carbon dioxide transported to the lungs for elimination.

Above the *anaerobic threshold,* lactic acid released from working muscle diffuses into the blood where it combines with bicarbonate ions:

$$H^+\text{-lactate} + HCO_3^- \longleftrightarrow H_2O + CO_2 + \text{lactate}$$

As plasma bicarbonate ions are consumed, carbon dioxide released from this reaction is eliminated in the lungs along with the carbon dioxide generated by normal aerobic metabolism. A decrease in the plasma bicarbonate concentration at normal P_{CO_2} causes a fall in arterial pH, which is detected by the peripheral chemoreceptors. This arterial acidosis stimulates ventilation out of proportion to the level of exercise intensity. As the acidosis becomes more severe the increased ventilation causes a decrease in alveolar and arterial P_{CO_2} (see Chapter 9).

ABNORMAL BREATHING PATTERNS

In some disease states, the pattern of breathing can become significantly altered. Figure 8–8 shows two examples of altered breathing patterns seen commonly. *Cheyne-Stokes* ventilation is characterized by a varying tidal volume and ventilatory frequency. Following a period of apnea, tidal volume and frequency increase progressively over several breaths. This activity then decreases until another period of apnea is seen. This irregular breathing pattern is seen in some patients who sustain traumatic head injury or who develop other central nervous system dysfunction. It is also seen occasionally in normal subjects during sleep at high altitude. The mechanism responsible for Cheyne-Stokes ventilation is not fully understood. Under conditions in which brain blood flow is low, it may involve feedback oscillation of the respiratory control center caused by a delay in the transit of blood from the lungs to the brain. In other circumstances it may involve neural oscillation in the respiratory control centers arising from focal tissue injury.

Apneustic breathing is another abnormal breathing pattern (see Figure 8–8). It is characterized by sustained periods of inspiration separated by brief periods of expiration. This ventilatory pattern is sometimes seen in patients with central nervous system injury. It is believed to be caused by loss of inspiratory-inhibitory activity that results in a relatively augmented inspiratory drive.

Altered breathing patterns are also commonly seen during sleep, where brief episodes of apnea or hyperventilation occur. In healthy individuals the apnea episodes are usually brief and do not cause significant arterial hypercapnia (increased P_{CO_2}) or arterial hypoxemia. However, in *sleep apnea syndromes* the duration of apnea is abnormally prolonged, causing significant increases in arterial P_{CO_2} and decreases in arterial hemoglobin saturation.

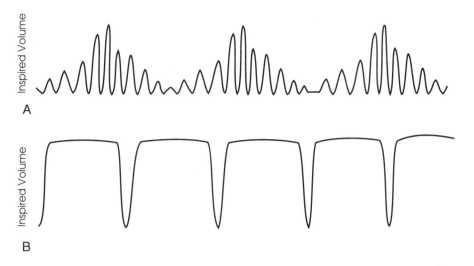

A

B

Figure 8–8. Abnormal breathing patterns. *A.* Cheyne-Stokes respiration is characterized by periods of waxing and waning ventilatory activity separated by periods of no ventilatory activity (apnea). *B.* Apneustic breathing is characterized by sustained deep inspirations, separated by short periods of exhalation.

The most common form of sleep apnea is *obstructive sleep apnea,* which occurs when the upper airway (usually the hypopharynx) closes during inspiration. This can occur when the intra-airway pressure decreases at the start of inspiration, causing the hypopharynx to be pulled shut (usually at the base of the tongue). This is similar in mechanism to the process of snoring, but is more extreme because it occludes the airway and stops inspiration. Patients with obstructive sleep apnea are aroused by the respiratory drive arising from chemoreceptor activity generated when the hypoxemia and hypercapnia become severe. When this occurs, respiration is restored briefly, until another apneic episode occurs. This cycle can repeat itself many times per hour and cause significant sleep deprivation even though the patient does not awaken fully and is unaware of the process. Causes of obstructive sleep apnea include obesity, excessive compliance of the hypopharynx, edema in the upper airway, and structural abnormalities of the upper airways. In *central sleep apnea* the cause of breathing cessation is a decrease in ventilatory drive to the respiratory motor neurons. Mixed forms of central and obstructive sleep apnea are commonly seen. Obstructive sleep apnea can be treated using devices worn by the patient that pull the tongue forward during sleep (to prevent its compression of the hypopharynx). Alternatively, air can be delivered by a nasal mask to increase the pressure in the upper airways during sleep, preventing collapse (nasal continuous positive pressure ventilation).

Chapter 9

Physiology of Exercise

The lung functions continuously to maintain a narrow range of oxygenation (near full saturation) and partial pressure of carbon dioxide (36 to 44 torr) in the blood. Thus far, the physiological properties of the lung in accomplishing its gas exchange function have been considered only in the resting state. However, the moment-to-moment metabolic demands of the body vary enormously, and significant increases in metabolism are associated with the muscular work of exercise. The assessment of exercise performance is of particular interest in clinical medicine because it is sometimes difficult or impossible to assess the cause of breathlessness or symptoms of exercise limitation from quiescent tests of pulmonary function.

The *cardiovascular system* must increase circulation of blood for increased oxygen delivery for energy production and increased disposal of the metabolic product of work (carbon dioxide). This is accomplished by increasing cardiac output and redistributing blood flow, predominantly to skeletal muscle. Ultimately, exercise intensity is limited by the ability of the cardiovascular system to accomplish this function.

The *musculoskeletal system* facilitates skeletal muscle contraction by the bioenergetic conversion of chemical energy stored as glucose into kinetic energy.

The *central nervous system* must deliver coordinated impulses to the musculoskeletal system to trigger muscle contraction in appropriate muscle groups. Failure of this system to function properly leads to impaired exercise capacity by causing muscle weakness (e.g., as in multiple sclerosis, poliomyelitis, or amyotrophic lateral sclerosis). The central nervous system also controls that intangible component of superlative exercise performance — motivation. The *autonomic nervous system* is important in regulating the visceral component of exercise — accelerating heart rate and redistributing blood flow among organs to meet the requirements of dynamic exercise.

The *respiratory system* receives blood flow equal to the entire cardiac output. At rest, this system need not function very efficiently, because it is not working near its maximum capacity. In normal individuals, the gas exchange capability of the respiratory system *never* is the limiting factor in exercise. Energy production during endurance exercise and oxygen transport (in maximal exercise) limit exercise in normal persons. However, when lung gas exchange is impaired, it may become the limiting factor in exercise performance.

Bioenergetics

During exercise, oxygen consumption can increase from about 250 ml/min to 3000 ml/min or more. During exercise, the consumption of oxygen ($\dot{V}o_2$) is proportional to the exercise intensity. Skeletal muscle contracts as the result of the cross-bridge formation between myosin and actin, which results from the hydrolysis of adenosine triphosphate (ATP). In skeletal muscle, ATP is not stored in great quantities; rather, the high-energy phosphate bond is stored as creatine phosphate (CP). It is converted quickly, as needed, to ATP from the available stores by the following reaction:

$$CP + ADP \xrightarrow{\text{creatine phosphokinase}} creatine + ATP$$

ATP is produced by aerobic and anaerobic metabolism of carbohydrate. Other potential energy sources include fats and protein. Fat cannot be metabolized anaerobically. As exercise intensity increases, fat is less utilized. At maximal exercise there is a marked increase in utilization of glucose and a marked decrease in utilization of fats for energy production. Because glucose stores are limited, this imposes a limitation to exercise endurance. The body stores an average of 200,000 kilocalories (kcal) in fat but only 2,000 kcal as carbohydrate (mostly as glycogen). During endurance exercise (e.g., during marathon running), these stores may be entirely depleted — the infamous "wall" that runners reach

around the 20-mile mark. Protein is not metabolized for energy production either at rest or during exercise; gluconeogenesis from protein occurs significantly only during starvation states when other energy stores are depleted.

At rest, both fat and carbohydrate are metabolized equally according to the following equations:

Carbohydrate:

$$\underbrace{C_6H_{12}O_6}_{\text{glucose}} + \underbrace{6O_2 \longrightarrow 6CO_2}_{RQ = 1.0} + 6H_2O + 36 \text{ ATP}$$

$$\sim P : O_2 = 6.0$$

Fat:

$$\underbrace{C_{16}H_{32}O_6}_{\text{palmitate}} + \underbrace{23O_2 \longrightarrow 16CO_2}_{RQ = 0.71} + 16H_2O + 130 \text{ ATP}$$

$$\sim P : O_2 = 5.65$$

The *respiratory quotient* (RQ) is the ratio of carbon dioxide molecules produced to oxygen molecules consumed. During exercise, the RQ increases with the level of exercise intensity, reflecting a change in the utilization of substrates from fat to carbohydrate. The *respiratory exchange ratio* (R) is the value of the RQ measured from lung gas exchange at the mouth. During steady state, the R must equal the RQ. Note that the RQ is different for carbohydrate (1.0) and fat (~ 0.7). At rest, the RQ is approximately 0.85, which reflects a balance between fat and glucose oxidation. During progressively increasing exercise, the RQ increases toward 1.0. This reflects a shift from fat to glucose metabolism. A physiological consequence of this shift from utilization of fat and carbohydrate to more predominant glucose metabolism is the slightly increased oxygen utilization that is required to produce ATP. When glucose alone is metabolized, 6.0 ATP molecules containing high energy phophate bonds ($\sim P$) are produced for each oxygen molecule consumed. When a molecule of fat is metabolized, the ratio is about 5.65 oxygen molecules per $\sim P$. A physiological disadvantage of increased carbohydrate utilization is the increased amount of carbon dioxide production per mole of ATP produced. This results from the increased RQ of glucose metabolism versus fat metabolism. Thus, relative to glucose, metabolism of fat requires somewhat more oxygen for equivalent energy production but causes relatively less production of carbon dioxide per mole of ATP produced.

The quantitative measure of exercise intensity is oxygen consumption ($\dot{V}O_2$) defined as the volume of oxygen consumed per unit of time (ml/min). As energy demands increase, the capacity to produce ATP solely by aerobic metabolism is exceeded and anaerobic metabolism ensues. Normally, this occurs at about 50% of maximal oxygen consumption ($\dot{V}O_{2max}$). Above the point where anaerobic metabolism begins, oxygen is still consumed, and ATP is produced by *two* pathways. Aerobic metabolism continues and increases further with increased tissue demand for ATP, and anaerobic metabolism begins and adds to the production of ATP. During anaerobic metabolism:

$$C_6H_{12}O_6 \longrightarrow 2\ C_3H_6O_3 + 2\ ATP$$
$$\text{Glucose} \qquad\quad \text{Lactic acid}$$

The lactic acid that is formed anaerobically in the muscle cells enters the blood and is dissociated almost completely at the pH of body fluids. It is buffered predominantly by the carbonic acid–bicarbonate system:

$$CH_3CHOHCOO^-H^+ + NaHCO_3 \longrightarrow$$
$$\text{Lactic acid} \qquad\qquad \text{Bicarbonate}$$

$$CH_3CHOHCOONa + H_2CO_3$$
$$\text{Sodium lactate} \qquad \text{Carbonic acid}$$

In the plasma, carbonic acid dissociates into water and carbon dioxide:

$$H_2CO_3 \longrightarrow H_2O + CO_2$$

Note that carbon dioxide formed from this buffering reaction comes from the decrease in plasma bicarbonate. Anaerobic metabolism is not nearly as efficient as aerobic metabolism for energy production because only 2 ATP molecules are produced per molecule of glucose consumed. In aerobic metabolism, 36 ATP molecules are produced from each glucose molecule.

Anaerobic threshold is defined as the point at which lactate production can be detected. Thus, it is the point at which lactate begins to accumulate in the blood. This leads to development of a metabolic

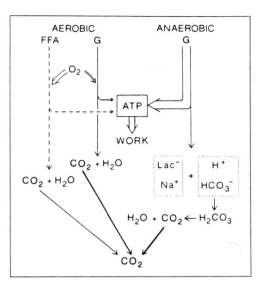

Figure 9–1. Aerobic and anaerobic pathways of substrate utilization in exercising muscle. Thickness of arrows of the reaction routes (substrate utilization, oxygen consumption, carbon dioxide production) is proportional to rates of flux of substrate per unit of adenosine triphosphate (ATP) production. G, glucose; FFA, free fatty acid. (From Ward SA, Davis JA, Whipp BJ: The physiologic basis of exercise testing: Principles, J Cardiovasc Pulmonary Tech 10:23–30, 1992.)

acidosis. In compensating for this, the respiratory control system increases the minute ventilation, causing a compensatory respiratory alkalosis (see Chapter 8). Figure 9–1 shows the pathways of energy production and substrate utilization. Note that anaerobic metabolism utilizes only glucose. Thus, anaerobic metabolism depletes glucose stores exclusively. Anaerobic metabolism also produces much less ATP for the same level of glucose consumption.

Muscle Fiber Types

Table 9–1 shows some of the various fiber types found in human skeletal muscle. Each is adapted for a specific type of exercise. Slow oxidative fibers develop active tension less quickly than other fiber types, and they are termed *slow-twitch* fibers. These fibers are better suited for oxidative metabolism than are *fast-twitch* fibers, which have a greater glycolytic capacity. Because slow-twitch fibers have a greater ability to utilize oxidative metabolism, maximal exercise in these fibers is accompanied by

TABLE 9-1
Skeletal Muscle Fiber Classification

Characteristics	Type I Slow Oxidative	Type IIA Fast Oxidative	Type IIB Fast Oxidative
"Color"	Red	Red	White
Myoglobin content	High	High	Low
Triglyceride content	High	Moderate	Low
Glycogen content	No appreciable differences		
Glycolytic capacity	Moderate	High	High
Oxidative potential (mitochondrial content, oxidative enzyme potential, capillary density)	High	High	Low
Fiber diameter	Moderate	Small	Large
Contractile behavior (time to peak tension following activation, myosin ATPase rate)	Slow	Fast	Fast

"delayed" anaerobiasis relative to fast-twitch fibers. Hence, slow-twitch fibers are more suited to types of activity requiring endurance. Marathon runners, for example, have a higher content of slow-twitch fibers in their vastus muscles than do olympic kayakers, whereas kayakers have a higher content of slow-twitch fibers in their deltoid muscles. Specific forms of training may alter the distribution of slow-twitch fibers in an adaptive manner to augment endurance exercise performance.

CARDIOVASCULAR FUNCTION IN EXERCISE

Exercise is both facilitated and limited by the capacity of the cardiovascular system to deliver oxygen to skeletal muscle. The cardiac output is generated as the product of the heart rate and the stroke volume. In a normal adult, resting heart rate can treble (e.g., from 70 to 210 beats per minute) and stroke volume can double so that an overall increase in cardiac output by sixfold is possible (Table 9–2). With training, stroke volume increases and heart rate slows at any level of exercise. However, maximal heart rate, which essentially is dictated by age, remains the same. Therefore, if the conditioned athlete has a resting heart rate of 45 and this increases to 210, heart rate is increased by four and one-half times; if stroke volume is doubled, cardiac output increases ninefold in maximal exercise. It is this acquired cardiac conditioning and increased maximal cardiac output that results in the improved athletic performance with training.

Dynamic control of the cardiovascular system during exercise is regulated by the autonomic nervous system. Parasympathetic activity to the heart decreases, and sympathetic neural activity increases. Heart rate increases even before exercise is begun, indicating the anticipatory linkage between consciousness (central motivation) and autonomic activity. Shortly after exercise begins, circulating catecholamines (predominantly epinephrine) further augment the increase in heart rate (as demonstrated by the slight increase in heart rate seen during exercise in patients with cardiac transplants). Epinephrine also augments the mobilization of glucose from glycogen stores. Sympathetically mediated vasoconstriction also contributes to the increased venous return of blood, which normally is pooled to a degree in the venous system. Venous return is further augmented physically by the contraction of exercising muscles. Finally, increased

TABLE 9–2
Normal Cardiovascular Response to Exercise

Parameter	Effect of Maximal Exercise
Heart rate	Threefold increase
Stroke volume	Twofold increase
Cardiac output (heart rate × stroke volume)	Sixfold increase
Blood pressure	Increases to 210 torr systolic; diastolic changes little
Skeletal muscle blood flow	Increases from 15% to 80% of total cardiac output
Renal and central nervous system blood flow	Remain constant due to increased blood pressure, but do not increase during exercise
Sympathetic neural activity	Increases causing: Increased venous return; Increased stroke volume; Increased blood pressure; Increased heart rate
Parasympathetic activity	Decreases, resulting in diminished activity in "nonessential" organs

venous return distends the left ventricle of the heart to a more favorable point on its length–tension curve. This elicits a stronger contraction (increased stroke volume) with each beat.

A major consequence (and requirement) of exercise is the redistribution of blood flow away from the viscera toward working skeletal muscle. At rest, about 15% to 20% of the cardiac output is distributed to skeletal muscle; during exercise, this can increase to 80%. However, adequate blood flow is still maintained in nonmuscular tissues by local autoregulation of blood flow. The vasodilation of arterioles in working muscles results from local release of metabolic vasodilators in these tissues caused by metabolic events of exercise. Blood pressure increases during exercise, especially systolic pressure, which may reach 210 torr. This facilitates the redistribution of blood flow away from resting tissues toward working skeletal muscle. Diastolic pressure changes only minimally, if at all.

RESPIRATORY FUNCTION IN EXERCISE

During rest, the lung utilizes only a small portion of its ventilatory capacity to meet metabolic demands.

However, during exercise, minor abnormalities in lung oxygenation or significant abnormalities in pulmonary mechanical properties (obstruction or restriction) may become limiting factors in the level of exercise that can be sustained. The arterial blood pH, Po_2, and Pco_2 remain nearly constant over a wide range of aerobic exercise in normal individuals. As the oxygen consumption ($\dot{V}o_2$) increases in exercise, carbon dioxide output ($\dot{V}co_2$) also increases. Accordingly, the alveolar ventilation must increase to eliminate this additional carbon dioxide or respiratory acidosis will occur. Above the anaerobic threshold, lactate begins to accumulate and pH begins to decrease. Figure 9–2 demonstrates the relationship between carbon dioxide production and the alveolar ventilation necessary to excrete carbon dioxide at each level of production. This figure indicates the minute ventilation necessary to maintain a particular $Paco_2$ at a $\dot{V}co_2$ of 2 liters/min, which is achieved with moderate exercise. Note that to maintain a $Paco_2$ of 50 torr at this level of carbon dioxide production, the alveolar ventilation ($\dot{V}A$) need be only 38 liters/min. To maintain a $Paco_2$ of 30 torr, $\dot{V}A$ must be increased to 60 liters/min (i.e., increased by more than 50%). For the patient with chronic obstructive pulmonary disease,

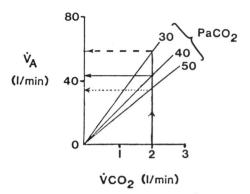

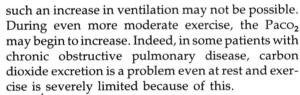

Figure 9-2. Alveolar ventilation required for a $\dot{V}CO_2$ of 2 liters/min (moderate exercise). Isopleths indicate the corresponding level of alveolar ventilation ($\dot{V}A$) necessary to maintain a $PaCO_2$ of 50, 40, or 30 torr. (From Leff AR [ed]: Cardiopulmonary Exercise Testing, Orlando, FL, Grune & Stratton, 1986.)

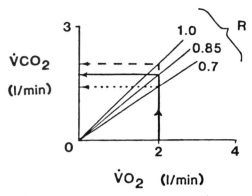

Figure 9-3. Carbon dioxide production ($\dot{V}CO_2$) for a $\dot{V}O_2$ of 2 liters/min (moderate exercise). Isopleths are for respiratory equivalents (R) of 0.7, 0.85, and 1.0. (From Leff AR [ed]: Cardiopulmonary Exercise Testing, Orlando, FL, Grune & Stratton, 1986.)

such an increase in ventilation may not be possible. During even more moderate exercise, the $PaCO_2$ may begin to increase. Indeed, in some patients with chronic obstructive pulmonary disease, carbon dioxide excretion is a problem even at rest and exercise is severely limited because of this.

As $\dot{V}O_2$ increases during progressively greater exercise intensity, the R increases toward 1.0, reflecting the increased production of carbon dioxide. Figure 9-3 compares the required level of carbon dioxide excretion ($\dot{V}CO_2$) for a $\dot{V}O_2$ of 2.0 liters/min for different levels of R. If fat alone were metabolized, the R would equal 0.7, and the $\dot{V}CO_2$ would be 1.4 liters/min. When only glucose is metabolized (the case at maximal exercise), the $\dot{V}CO_2$ is 2.0. Thus, when different substrates are used (glucose vs. fat) to achieve the same $\dot{V}O_2$, an increase of 0.6 liter/

min or about 43% more carbon dioxide is produced. Figure 9-3 also highlights the advantage gained with slow-twitch fibers, which utilize oxidative metabolism to a greater degree than fast-twitch fibers. For endurance exercise, these slow-twitch fibers can achieve a greater $\dot{V}O_2$ before reaching the anaerobic threshold.

Ventilation–Perfusion Relationships During Exercise

In Chapter 7, the normal, mild inhomogeneity of ventilation–perfusion was discussed. Figure 9-4A (left) shows a narrow dispersion of the $\dot{V}A/\dot{Q}$ around a mean $\dot{V}/\dot{Q}$ ratio; in this case the log standard deviation of blood flow = 0.6. In Figure 9-4B, a bimodal distribution is shown (log standard deviation of blood flow = 2.0). Such abnormal distribu-

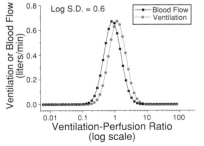

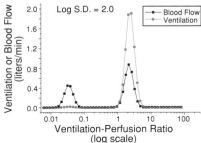

Figure 9-4. Distribution of ventilation–perfusion ratios in normal lung *(left)* and lung of patient with chronic obstructive pulmonary disease *(right)*.

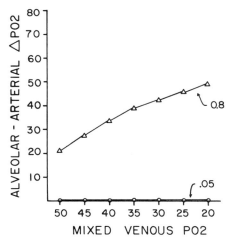

Figure 9–5. Effect of increased oxygen extraction on alveolar-arterial P_{O_2}. For a lung with a narrow distribution of ventilation–perfusion ratios (log S.D. = 0.05), progressive decrease in the mixed venous O_2 caused by increased extraction during exercise does not affect the alveolar-arterial P_{O_2}. For the lung of a patient with chronic obstructive pulmonary disease with a wide distribution of ventilation–perfusion (log S.D. = 0.8), increased extraction causes a progressive widening of the alveolar-arterial P_{O_2}. (From Leff AR [ed]: Cardiopulmonary Exercise Testing, Orlando, FL, Grune & Stratton, 1986.)

tions of $\dot{V}_A/\dot{Q}$ commonly occur in patients with asthma, chronic bronchitis, or interstitial lung disease.

In individuals with lung disease such as asthma or interstitial lung disease, exercise causes an increase in the alveolar-arterial oxygen difference ($[A - a]D_{O_2}$). Increased oxygen extraction during exercise further exacerbates the situation. With the progressive decrease in the $P\bar{v}_{O_2}$ that results from increased oxygen extraction with increasing exercise, there is a progressive increase in ($[A - a]D_{O_2}$). Thus, with exercise, patients with lung diseases may experience a decrease in Pa_{O_2} (Figure 9–5).

For normal patients having a narrow distribution of $\dot{V}_A/\dot{Q}$, increasing systemic oxygen extraction does not cause hypoxemia. Lung units having very poor $\dot{V}_A/\dot{Q}$, such as those occurring in disease states, do not exist in normal subjects, and there is no oxygen desaturation in arterial blood, even with the most severe levels of exercise (see Figure 9–5).

Mechanical Limitations to Respiration in Exercise

The maximal ventilation that can be sustained for 1 minute is termed the *maximal ventilatory capacity*

(MVC). This capacity (= volume) is equal to about 40 times the forced expiratory volume in 1 second (FEV_1) in normal subjects. The maximal ventilation that can be sustained for a prolonged period of work is only about 60% of the MVC in normal individuals because respiratory muscle fatigue otherwise will occur.

In disease states, exercise can be limited by the mechanical properties of the abnormal lung. In interstitial fibrosis, the lung is stiffer and thus harder to stretch on inspiration; these individuals also have an increased anatomical and physiological dead space that results from destruction of alveolar capillary beds. Because of the increased dead space, persons with pulmonary fibrosis must increase minute ventilation more to excrete the same amount of carbon dioxide than normal individuals for a given level of exercise ($\dot{V}_{O_2}$). Patients with pulmonary fibrosis may use more than 80% of their MVC during maximal exercise. However, unlike normal individuals having lungs of normal compliance, these patients must also overcome the increased elastance of their lungs. During exercise, normal individuals increase minute ventilation first by increasing tidal volume (V_T). After a twofold increase in tidal volume, respiratory rate then begins to increase and causes the needed increase in total ventilation ($\dot{V}_E$) to execute the incremental production of carbon dioxide. When lung or chest wall elastance is increased substantially in restrictive diseases, the work of breathing becomes great, and respiratory muscle fatigue may ensue. To minimize the work of breathing, patients with pulmonary fibrosis increase $\dot{V}_E$ during exercise by increasing ventilatory rate rather than tidal volume at the beginning of exercise.

Subjects with obstructive airways disease also have more limited ventilatory capacity than normal subjects. This is because of the high resistance to airflow, which increases the work of breathing, especially at high respiratory rates. Accordingly, these individuals increase $\dot{V}_E$ during exercise by increasing V_T without increasing respiratory rate, which is limited by the prolonged time required for expiration (Figure 9–6).

PHYSIOLOGICAL EXERCISE TESTING

There are many ways by which exercise performance can be assessed in human subjects. All of these

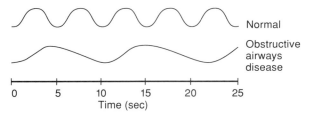

Figure 9–6. Tidal breathing pattern in normal patient *(top)* and patient with obstructive pulmonary disease *(bottom)*. In patient with increased airway resistance, both inspiration and (especially) expiration are prolonged. This limits the frequency of respiration with increased ventilatory demand during exercise.

methods must relate the $\dot{V}o_2$, which is the absolute index of exercise intensity, to other physiological parameters. Figure 9–7 shows the apparatus used for *graded exercise testing*. The subject is seated on a bicycle ergometer, and a mouthpiece is inserted to measure gas flows and concentrations during inspiration and expiration. A *pneumotachograph* inserted into this circuit measures flow, which is integrated into volume both on a breath-by-breath basis and cumulatively. The subject is instructed to pedal, and by application of a braking mechanism, the work of pedaling becomes progressively more difficult. The power output (watts) is increased in a stepwise manner at approximately 1-minute intervals after

an initial period of unloaded pedaling. Note that with 1-minute increments, true steady state is never achieved. Nonetheless, this enables measurement of exercise performance at multiple stages from rest to maximum. The subject is coached vigorously to complete the highest level of exercise (*maximal exercise* = the greatest $\dot{V}o_2$) possible as the power load is increased. Figure 9–8 is a schematic representation of the exercise performance of a normal individual. Note that $\dot{V}o_2$ increases linearly with power output (workload). Heart rate also increases linearly until the maximal rate is achieved (not shown). Maximum heart rate is age-related and decreases with age. As exercise intensity increases, R increases toward a ratio of 1.0. However, substrate metabolism does not define anaerobic threshold. The anaerobic threshold is defined by lactate production. When lactate is produced in excess of the ability to the blood to buffer it, arterial blood pH decreases. This decrease in arterial blood pH elicits an increase in $\dot{V}e$. At the anaerobic threshold, the relationship between $\dot{V}e$ and $\dot{V}o_2$ increases sharply from its slope at lesser $\dot{V}o_2$. The new $\dot{V}e$ slope has two phases. First it parallels the increased $\dot{V}co_2$, which results from the increased production of carbon dioxide from lactate buffering during and aerobic metabolism. Later, a steeper slope in $\dot{V}e$ occurs.

The first increase in $\dot{V}e$ is somewhat less than the subsequent increase. During the first period, the

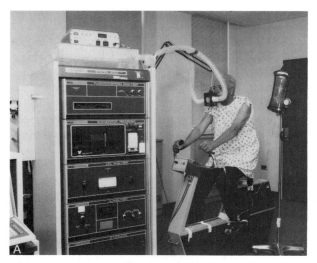

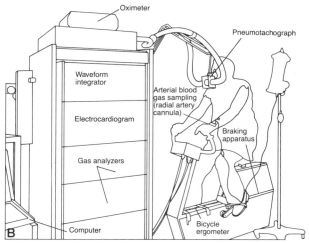

Figure 9–7. *A* and *B*. Apparatus for clinical assessment of dynamic exercise physiology.

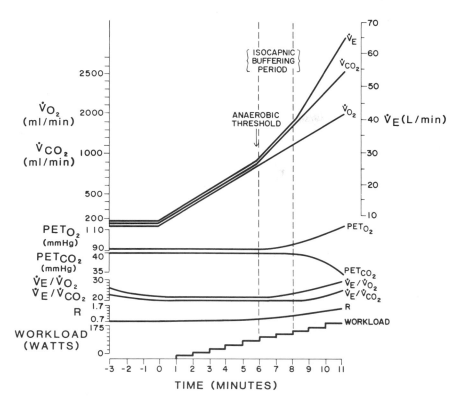

Figure 9–8. Schematic tracing of some important parameters during ramped dynamic exercise test. See text for discussion. Compare with actual tracing in Figure 9–9. Abbreviations are in text. (From Leff AR [ed]: Cardiopulmonary Exercise Testing, Orlando, FL, Grune & Stratton, 1986.)

blood pH decreases to about 7.32 to 7.34, but the chemoreceptor response is less than in the next period. This first phase is referred to as the period of *isocapnic buffering*. After about 2 minutes of increasing exercise, the chemoreceptor stimulation of ventilation increases, but the arterial blood pH still remains below 7.35.

Note that the partial pressure of end-tidal oxygen (P_{ETO_2}) begins to increase during the isocapnic period, but the partial pressure of end-tidal carbon dioxide (P_{ETCO_2}) does not decrease until the end of the period. At the start of the isocapnic buffering period, ventilation is stimulated by the increased $\dot{V}_{CO_2}$ arising from the buffering of lactate acid by bicarbonate. This increase in $\dot{V}_E$ is out of proportion to the $\dot{V}_{O_2}$, so alveolar (and end-tidal) P_{O_2} increases. At the end of the isocapnic buffering period, acidosis stimulates ventilation out of proportion to *both* $\dot{V}_{O_2}$ and $\dot{V}_{CO_2}$, so end-tidal P_{O_2} rises further and end-tidal P_{CO_2} decreases. Since the anaerobic threshold (AT) is defined as the first point at which excess lactate production occurs, the point where

P_{ETO_2} first increases is an excellent noninvasive measure of AT. Technically, the best way to measure AT would be to measure blood lactate in multiple samples. This has been done, and it has been shown that the P_{ETO_2} corresponds closely to the point where blood lactate increases during graded, non-steady-state exercise.

Curves similar to those obtained for the P_{ETO_2} and P_{ETCO_2} are obtained by dividing the $\dot{V}_E$ at a given level of exercise by the $\dot{V}_{O_2}$ or $\dot{V}_{CO_2}$ to obtain the ratios $\dot{V}_E/\dot{V}_{O_2}$ and $\dot{V}_E/\dot{V}_{O_2}$. Termed *ventilatory equivalents for oxygen and carbon dioxide*, comparison of these indices more clearly demonstrates the onset of AT (see Figure 9–8). Note that the $\dot{V}_E/\dot{V}_{O_2}$ curve gives the same information as the P_{ETO_2} curve in assessing anaerobic threshold.

Figure 9–9 is an actual tracing from a ramped exercise test. In assessing exercise performance, some measures are particularly important. Foremost is the maximal level of exercise that can be achieved, as measured by the $\dot{V}_{O_2}$ ($\dot{V}_{O_{2max}}$). Even where this is relatively normal, however, other

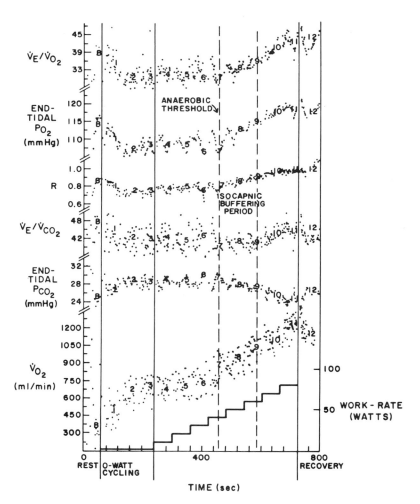

Figure 9–9. Actual tracing from a normal subject during exercise. Numbers on each tracing correspond to minutes of exercise. Each point is a calculation derived from instantaneous sampling of a single expired breath. (From Leff AR [ed]: Cardiopulmonary Exercise Testing, Orlando, FL, Grune & Stratton, 1986.)

aspects of abnormal performance still may be assessed. If $\dot{V}E$ is increased initially by accelerating respiratory rate rather than tidal volume, this suggests increased lung elastance and a possible pulmonary restrictive process (see earlier). Normally, the anaerobic threshold occurs at about 50% of the $\dot{V}_{O_{2max}}$. Where the anaerobic threshold occurs at significantly less than 50% of maximal $\dot{V}_{O_2}$, this suggests either poor cardiac conditioning or cardiac failure. Cardiac performance may also be assessed by calculating the ratio of maximal $\dot{V}_{O_2}$/maximal heart rate. This ratio, the O_2-pulse, is a reflection of the effective stroke volume of the heart. If an especially rapid rate is required to achieve an expected $\dot{V}_{O_2}$, the amount of blood ejected with each heart-beat is relatively reduced, and O_2-pulse is reduced from normal levels. A decreased O_2-pulse indicates either poor cardiac conditioning or, where reduced substantially, heart failure.

SUPRANORMAL EXERCISE

The study of exercise performance has implications in health as well as in diagnosis of disease. A reasonable program of exercise, geared to the daily needs of an individual, may be helpful in facilitating maintenance of a healthy body weight and healthy cardiovascular conditioning. Exercise beyond this point is accomplished at a cost. History records that the first marathon was completed by a Greek runner, who on traversing the more than 26-mile distance, announced: "Victory is ours"! He then collapsed and died. Exceptionally rigorous exercise regimens are accompanied by injuries varying from minor symptoms of joint stress, to bone fractures, and, occasionally, to reproductions of the original marathon performance. Beyond levels that induce normal levels of cardiovascular conditioning, exercise produces no incremental health benefit. There is a potential for compulsive exercisers to cause themselves harm.

Part II

Chapter 10

Lung Growth and Development

The process of growth and development of the respiratory system is a continuous maturational phenomenon. Prior to birth, respiratory functions occurring in utero are mediated by placental diffusion. The lungs are nonfunctional, and the fetus has no direct gas exchange with the external environment. At birth, the neonate must, within a brief moment, expand its lungs and begin an entirely different form of respiration — direct exchange of gas with the atmosphere. Although lung development is far from complete and differentiation continues into the eighth year of postnatal life, the newly born air-breathing neonate must be able to transport oxygen, excrete carbon dioxide, and defend the internal environment of the lung from the environmental insults from which it was sheltered during fetal life.

RESPIRATION BEFORE BREATHING

The fetus is well adapted to its intrauterine environment. As for adults, the developing fetus requires oxygen for metabolism and excretes carbon dioxide as the product of metabolism. The weight-averaged metabolic rate of the fetus ($\dot{V}o_2$/kg body weight) is about twice that of the adult — reflecting the rapid growth and differentiation process that is occurring.

Blood from the uterine artery supplies the uterus and forms a large venous plexus in the uterus of the mother during pregnancy (Figure 10–1). The placenta is the organ of gas exchange for the fetus. Its microvilli interdigitate with the maternal uterine circulation and, by passive diffusion, the blood vessels of the fetal circulation take on oxygen from the

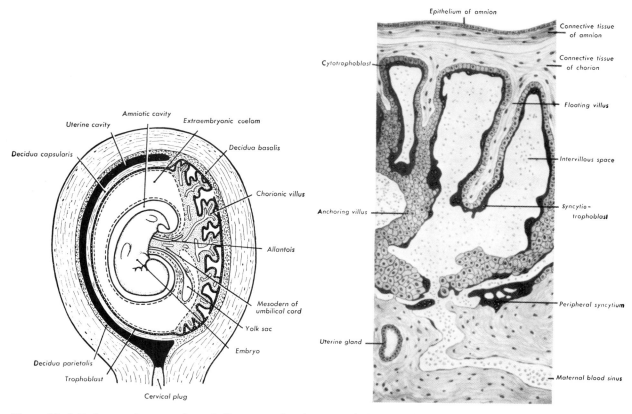

Figure 10–1. Exchange of gases and metabolites across the placenta. *Left.* Schema of the relationship between fetal and maternal circulation (gross structure). *Right.* Microstructure showing sinusoids that are the structures for gas exchange during fetal life. (From Copenhaven WD [ed]: Bailey's Textbook of Histology, 15th ed., Chap 20. © 1964, The Williams & Wilkins Co., Baltimore.)

maternal circulation and give up carbon dioxide to the maternal circulation. In the fetus, blood travels through the umbilical artery and, after gas exchange through the placenta, returns through the umbilical vein. The placenta is an outgrowth of the fetus, and the blood of the fetal and maternal circulations do not mix (see Figure 10–1). The uterus and the placenta each maintain a separate circulation. Because the uterus extracts oxygen to meet its own metabolic demands, the partial pressure of oxygen delivered to the fetus (PfaO_2) is relatively low compared with adult arterial oxygen tensions. Consider that the maternal PaO_2 is 95 to 100 torr. [Actually, it is generally a bit lower later in pregnancy, because the abdominal mass of the fetus compresses the diaphragm. This causes basilar atelectasis, which results in shunting through these regions and a reduc-

tion in the maternal PaO_2]. At the capillary level, the PO_2 in the uterine vein decreases to 40 torr, as the uterus itself is nourished. Note that the arterial oxygen of the fetus results from gas exchange with *venous* blood from the mother. The PO_2 in the umbilical vein thus is only 30 torr, and in the umbilical artery the PO_2 is only 20 torr (Figure 10–2).

How can a fetus grow and develop at oxygen tensions incompatible with adult life, especially when its metabolic demands are twice those of adult life? Perhaps the most important adaptation to this environment is the presence of fetal hemoglobin, which has a substantially greater affinity for oxygen than does adult hemoglobin. Consisting of two γ chains in place of the β chains of adult hemoglobin, fetal hemoglobin has a P_{50} of 20 torr versus the P_{50} of adult hemoglobin, which is 27 torr. Thus, there is

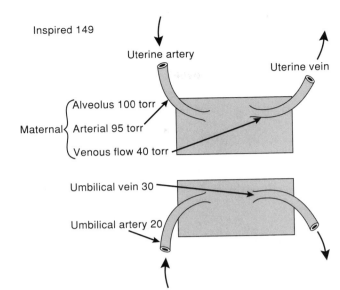

Figure 10–2. Schema of stepdown in the partial pressure of oxygen from the atmosphere to the fetal arterial circulation.

a rightward shift in the oxygen-hemoglobin dissociation curve of the adult relative to the fetus. Because the hemoglobin concentration is relatively increased in the fetus, fetal hemoglobin also has a much greater oxygen-carrying capacity than does adult hemoglobin (Figure 10–3). For example, at an arterial P_{O_2} of 20 torr, the Cf_{aO_2} is 12 ml/dl blood. At 100 torr, the maternal blood oxygen content is only 15 ml/dl. Thus, fetal arterial oxygen content is 75% of that of the mother, despite a P_{O_2} of 20 torr.

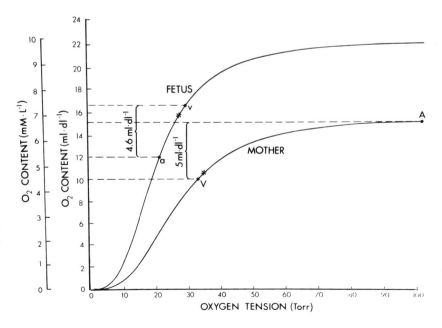

Figure 10–3. Oxygen–hemoglobin dissociation curves for adult (e.g., maternal) and fetal hemoglobin. Note the greater affinity of oxygen for fetal blood than for adult blood. At lesser Pa_{O_2} there is substantially greater saturation of fetal hemoglobin. In addition, the hemoglobin concentration in fetal blood is greater than in the mother. These differences result in a greater oxygen content in umbilical venous (fetal arterial) blood than in uterine venous blood. (Adapted from Longo LD: Respiration before birth: The placenta. In Scarpelli EM [ed]: Pulmonary Physiology: Fetus, Newborn, Child, Adolescent, 2nd ed. Philadelphia, Lea & Febiger, 1990. Reproduced with permission.)

ANATOMICAL DIFFERENTIATION

Development in Utero

The cells that form the respiratory tract develop from entodermally derived epithelium. These cells will form the tissues of the conducting airways and alveoli, which will become intimately associated with the pulmonary circulation for the function of gas exchange.

Table 10–1 outlines the time course of fetal lung development. By the end of the fourth week after conception, the early rudiments of a tracheoesophageal septum are evident and buds that will become the right and left mainstem bronchi appear. In the fifth and sixth weeks of development, buds for the various lobes of the lung appear and bronchopulmonary segments arise. The lung now begins to take on a lobulated appearance.

The thoracic cavity is enclosed in the pleural space by the eighth week of development. At week 8, the first of three major fetal developmental phases, the *pseudoglandular phase*, begins. Throughout fetal development, the lung is collapsed and is filled with a fluid that it secretes.

Pseudoglandular Phase. This phase occurs during weeks 8 to 16 and is characterized by the dichoto-

TABLE 10–1
Anatomical Development of the Lung

Time	Event
Prenatal	
Day 26	Tracheoesophageal septum develops.
Day 28	Buds of mainstem bronchi appear.
Day 33	Buds of lung lobes appear.
Day 41	Bronchopulmonary segments develop; lung becomes lobulated.
Day 52	Pleural cavity is closed.
Week 8	Pseudoglandular phase occurs.
Week 16	Canalicular phase occurs.
Week 24	Saccular phase occurs and continues until birth.
BIRTH	
Postnatal	
2 months	Alveolar development begins.
2 years	Regular growth begins in place of septal formation.
7 years	Lung architecture is remodeled to adult pattern.
8 years	Alveolization ends; no further alveoli are formed during growth.
15 years	Normal growth is complete.

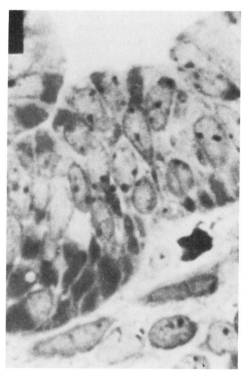

Figure 10–4. Formation of columnar airway epithelial cells at 8 weeks gestation (pseudoglandular phase). (Adapted from Snyder JM, Mendelson CR, Johnston JM: The morphology of lung development in the human fetus. In Nelson GH [ed]: Lung Biology in Health and Disease, vol. 27. New York, Marcel Dekker, 1985. Reproduced by courtesy of Marcel Dekker, Inc.)

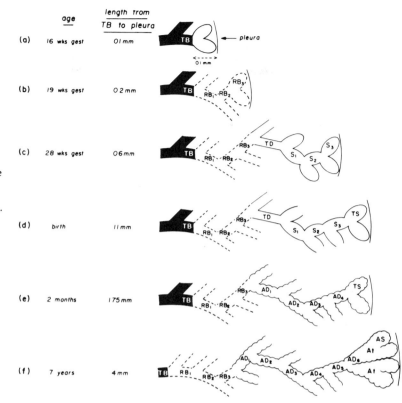

Figure 10–5. The process of alveolization. See text for description of each phase and also Table 10–1. (From Hislop A, Reid L: Development of the acinus in the human lung. Thorax 29:90, 1974.)

mous branching of the bronchial tree and development of the conducting airways. Approximately 23 to 27 generations of conducting airways are developed. These airways are lined by a columnar epithelium (Figure 10–4).

Canalicular Phase. During this phase there is a major proliferation of blood vessels as capillaries grow and move into close proximity to the tubules from which alveoli ultimately will develop. Epithelial cells now begin to show histological characteristics of type I and type II pneumocytes, and lamellar bodies that are associated with surfactant secretion can be found in type II cells (see later). There is also development and branching of the structures that will become the respiratory bronchioles.

Saccular Phase. During this phase which commences from week 24 to birth, the lung grows to fill the thoracic cavity and gas exchange units begin to develop. There is growth of peripheral ducts, and acinar development is completed prior to birth. In-

terestingly, there are relatively few alveoli at birth. The number of alveoli, which develop during the second month post partum, continues to increase to about 300 million by age 8 years, when growth is complete. Thus, gas exchange occurs at birth through the acini, as alveoli have not yet developed. Figure 10–5 shows the various stages of lung development and alveolization as the mature constituency of the lung is achieved.

MATERNAL ADAPTATIONS

The pregnant state imposes numerous physiological changes within the mother. Some of these are functional adaptations that clearly benefit fetal development. The massive growth of the uterus provides a safe environment for gestation. The enlarged and highly vascular uterus of pregnancy also provides nutritional and gas exchange functions during fetal development. In later stages of pregnancy, an adaptive cost is experienced by the mother. The average 15-kg weight gain occurs predominantly as the abdominal mass of the enlarged uterus. Increased production of progesterone during pregnancy stimulates respiration centrally, and both respiratory rate and tidal volume are increased. [The increase in total ventilation ($\dot{V}E$) caused by progesterone has been used therapeutically in nonpregnant patients who have primary disorders of ventilatory control that lead to alveolar hypoventilation. Supplemental administration of progesterone stimulates respiration in these individuals as well.]

The increase in $\dot{V}E$ causes a decrease in the arterial P_{CO_2} of the mother, and this persists throughout pregnancy. During pregnancy, uterine growth causes elevation of the diaphragm with changes in both the transverse diameter and the circumference. As a result, both expiratory reserve volume and functional residual capacity decrease, as is the case in all other states of abdominal mass or exogenous obesity. As the development continues, the intercostal muscles of the rib cage are used progressively more in inspiration.

The cardiac output increases substantially in the pregnant woman. At the 25th week of pregnancy, cardiac output may be increased as much as 40%, although by term it is only increased by about 15%. This important adaptation results from demands for placental nutrition. A placental blood flow murmur (bruit) can be heard during pregnancy; this results from the rapid flow caused by the functional arteriovenous shunt of the placenta. A pulmonic flow murmur is often heard during pregnancy. This is thought to be the result of decreased viscosity of the blood, another consequence of the "anemia of pregnancy," which is actually a dilutional hypervolemia.

Fetal Circulation and Respiration: Perinatal Events

The lung serves no respiratory function in utero. In adult life, the entire cardiac output passes through the systemic circulation. In fetal life, the venous return is diverted past the lung by passage through a patent *foramen ovale*, an opening in the atrial septum of the fetal heart. Venous blood entering the right ventricle is diverted to the systemic circulation through the ductus arteriosus (Figure 10–6). During fetal life, the pulmonary vascular resistance exceeds the systemic resistance; this is the consequence of hypoxic pulmonary vasoconstriction.

Accordingly, blood is shunted from the right atrium to the left atrium through the foramen ovale and diverted in part from the pulmonary artery to the thoracic aorta. There is no deleterious effect of this in utero, since respiration occurs through the placenta. Furthermore, this arrangement ensures that all regions of the developing lung (bronchial and pulmonary circulations) receive blood having arterial oxygen content.

At birth, several important events occur. Deprived of oxygen from the placental circulation, the neonate must expand its lungs. To do so, it must generate at least 30 cm H_2O inspiratory pressure. The process is abetted by the spreading of surfactant across the alveolar surface. Without surfactant, lung expansion is incomplete and collapsed lung regions persist. After lung inflation, the pulmonary vascular resistance decreases to one fifth of that in the systemic circulation, and blood flow is no longer diverted through the foramen ovale. The lung now begins to receive the full blood volume of the venous return. After several days, the ductus arteriosus closes. The mechanism by which this occurs is not understood fully but is thought to be related to the increased oxygen content of blood in the systemic circulation. The adult circulatory pattern is now established, but aspects of the fetal anatomy may persist. In some cases the ductus arteriosus does not close, necessitating surgical correction. The reflex of hypoxic vasoconstriction is not lost and may later (in adult life) influence lung gas exchange in disease states (see Chapter 4).

Under normal circumstances the transition from fetal to adult respiration occurs rapidly. The first phase occurs instantaneously at birth as the fetus takes its first breath. By 4 months of age, fetal hemoglobin is 90% replaced by adult hemoglobin, the ductus arteriosus is closed, and postnatal development of the infant proceeds into adult life.

Postnatal Development

As noted, alveolization continues until the eighth year of postnatal life. Alveolar septal formation is replaced by normal growth during the second through fifteenth years after birth. During life, both the volume of the lung parenchyma and the anatomical dead space increase in proportion to maturity. Figure 10–7 shows the development of the lung during life.

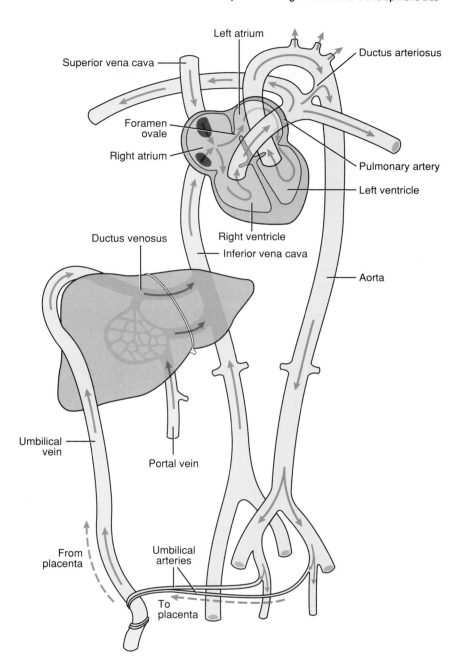

Figure 10-6. Fetal circulation. Note that blood is diverted away from the pulmonary circulation through the foramen ovale and ductus arteriosus. Both of these conduits close after birth when the pulmonary arterial blood pressure declines.

CELLULAR MORPHOGENESIS

Cells Derived from Entoderm

Secretory Cells. In larger airways, the secretory functions of the lung are subserved by goblet cells and serous cells. Together these cells create the secretions that determine the consistency of airway mucus that is essential to the trapping of foreign particulates and preservation of the sterile environment of the lung (see Chapter 11). *Goblet cells* are evident by the 13th week of gestation. They secrete neutral and acid mucus rich in sialic acid and con-

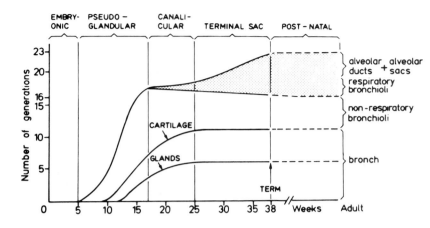

Figure 10-7. Chronology of lung development. (From Burri PH: Development and growth of the human lung. In Fishman AP, Fisher AB, Geiger SR [eds]: Handbook of Physiology, Section 3, The Respiratory System, vol 1. Bethesda, MD, American Physiological Society, 1985.)

tribute to the viscosity of mucus. *Serous cells* secrete neutral glycoproteins. They are present in the fetus but are absent in the adult except as a component of bronchial submucosal glands.

Bronchial glands are present only in conducting airways. They are derived from basal cells, which appear in the fetus by week 10 of gestation. Shortly after this time, bronchial mucus glands appear in the trachea. At the fourth month, these glands appear in the submucosa of the main bronchi. [Figure 12-8 shows schematically that these glands are located between the cartilage and surface epithelium.] They are complex structures consisting of ciliated cells at the orifice of the main duct and "nonspecified" cells in the collecting ducts of the glands. The secretory component consists of *mucus* cells near the distal end of the tubule and *serous* cells at the most distal end of the tubule (Figure 10-8).

Ciliated Cells. These cells line the conducting airways from the trachea to the respiratory bronchioles and are seen first in the 13th week of gestation. The mechanism by which ciliary action is initiated and coordinated is not fully understood. Throughout evolution the basic structural homology of these cells has been preserved; that is, they are similar in structure in protozoa and in mammals. In each cilium, the central dynein doublet is surrounded peripherally by nine single tubules. The central doublet contains an ATPase enzyme, and these tubules likely are responsible for the contractile beat of the cilium (Figure 10-9). Each epithelial

cell contains about 200 cilia, and a coordinated ciliary beat can be detected within the 13th week of gestation (the saccular phase).

Clara Cells. These cells develop at the bronchiolar level by the 16th week. They contain granules and so may have a secretory function; however, the precise product and function of these cells are not certain. Clara cells may also play a role in regeneration of the bronchial epithelium after injury.

Kulchitsky Cells. These cells are neuroendocrine cells that are similar to the argentaffin cells of the gastrointestinal tract. Technically they are not really of entodermal origin, since they are derived from neural crest cells. These cells appear in the fetus by week 15 and are more numerous in fetal than in adult life. They secrete biogenic amines including dopamine and 5-hydroxytryptamine (serotonin), but the functional significance of this is unclear. In a rare form of bronchial adenoma derived from this cell type, the *bronchial carcinoid tumor*, excessive neurohumoral secretion from these cells can lead to flushing (peripheral vasodilation) and anaphylactic reactions (hypotension). This tumor, which is far more common in the gastrointestinal tract, is believed to be derived from these cells.

Cells of the Alveoli. Three different cell types line the alveoli. The most prominent is the *type I pneu-*

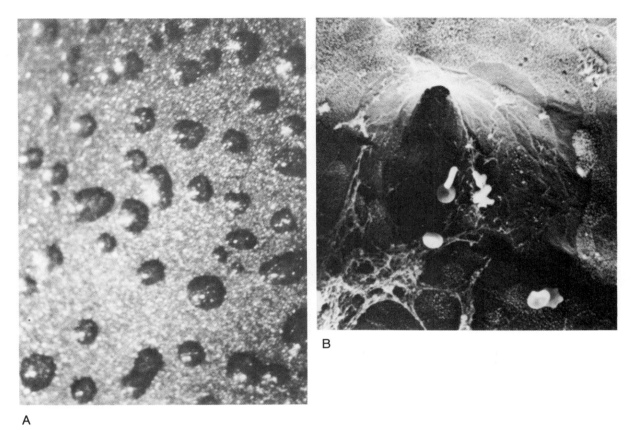

B

A

Figure 10–8. Identification of submucosal mucus secretion glands. *A.* The tracheal epithelium of the dog after parasympathetic stimulation. The little mounds are "hillocks" of mucus secreted from a single gland. *B.* Electron micrograph details the cone-shaped terminal portion of the mucus duct. (From Nadel JA: Control of airway muscle and secretion. Am Rev Respir Dis 115[6, part 2]:117–126, 1977. Reproduced with permission of the American Thoracic Society.)

mocyte. Yet this cell is only half as numerous as the *type II pneumocyte* (Figure 10–10). Shaped somewhat like a fried egg, the type I pneumocyte is spread thinly and flattened across the alveolar surface, so that it covers 95% of the alveolar surface area. Most gas exchange occurs through the thin processes of these cells (Figure 10–11). Type I cells are in close proximity to the endothelium of the capillary. *Type II pneumocytes* are the cells that secrete surfactant, the substance that reduces surface tension (Chapter 1). The spreading of surfactant on the alveolar surface is essential to the expansion of lungs in the neonate as the first breath is drawn and for normal life thereafter. Type III pneumocytes are also known as *brush cells.* These cells look like a hairbrush when viewed under scanning electron microscopy and can be found throughout the lung.

They are closely associated with nerves, and a chemoreceptor function for these cells has been postulated.

Cells Derived from Mesoderm

Smooth Muscle Cells. Smooth muscle cells differ substantially from both cardiac and striated cells. They contract and relax slowly and may shorten to very small lengths relative to their initial resting length. There are numerous gap junctions, which are assumed to be responsible for electrical coupling of these cells. Action potentials are not generated in airway smooth muscle, and there is no discrete sarcomeric organization involving Z-bands as is seen

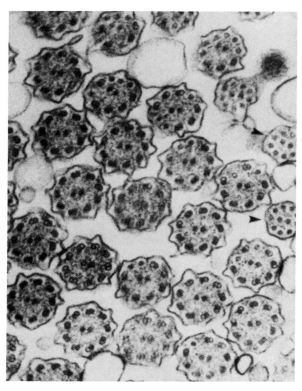

Figure 10–9. Electron photomicrograph of cilia from the trachea of a rabbit. Each cilium has two central tubules and nine peripheral tubules, a pattern of organization preserved through evolution from protozoa. (From Satir P, Dirksen ER: Function–structure correlations in cilia from mammalian respiratory tract. In Fishman AP, Fisher AB, Geiger SR [eds]: Handbook of Physiology, Section 3, The Respiratory System, vol 1. Bethesda, MD, American Physiological Society, 1985.)

for skeletal and cardiac muscle. Nonetheless, the contraction process occurs by the formation of actinomyosin cross-bridges. The details of the biology of airway smooth muscle are outlined in Chapter 12.

Airway smooth muscle develops in two discrete layers in the fetus. The inner layer is tangential, and the outer fibers travel longitudinally along the airway. This organization, which is similar to that of the gastrointestinal tract, is lost after early childhood. The functional significance of this maturational remodeling is uncertain, but there are major differences in the contractile response of airway smooth muscle that also occur during maturation. In adulthood, airway smooth muscle is organized in helical bundles around the bronchi. In the terminal airways, these cells become myelofibroblasts, which have contractile properties like airway smooth muscle cells. Airway smooth muscle cells of mesenchymal origin form by condensation around epithelial tubules beginning around the seventh week of gestation.

Pulmonary arteries have smooth muscle that resembles airway smooth muscle structurally, although the response to physiological and pharmacological stimulation differs completely between these tissues. The pulmonary arteries follow pathways taken by the airways, although there are at least five branching generations more for blood vessels than for airways. By the 14th gestational week, most of these pathways are developed. In

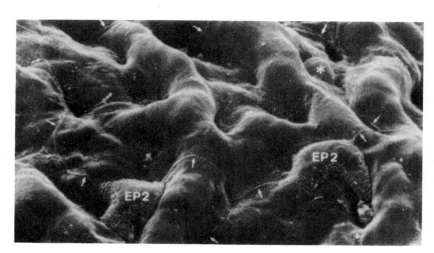

Figure 10–10. Scanning electron photomicrograph of alveolar type I pneumocyte (EP1) and type II (EP2) cells. Arrows show the boundaries of type I cell. (From Weibel ER: Design and structure of the human lung. In Fishman AP [ed]: Pulmonary Diseases and Disorders. New York, McGraw-Hill, 1980. Reproduced with permission of McGraw-Hill, Inc.)

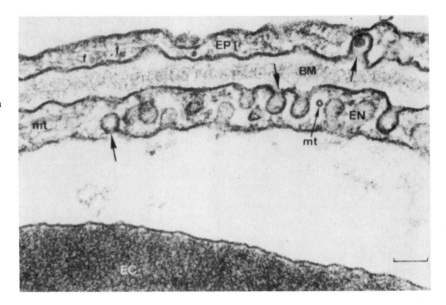

Figure 10–11. Interface between the endothelium of the capillary (EN) and a type I alveolocyte, across which gas exchange occurs. A single microtubule (mt) is seen. BM, basement membrane. Arrows show pinocytotic vesicles. (From Weibel ER: Lung cell biology. In Fishman AP, Fisher AB, Geiger SR [eds]: Handbook of Physiology, Section 3, The Respiratory System, vol 1. Bethesda, MD, American Physiological Society, 1985.)

contrast to the arteries, *pulmonary veins* follow the boundaries of the bronchopulmonary segments rather than the airways. The pulmonary veins are formed by evagination from the sinoatrial portion of the heart at the fifth week of fetal life.

The *vascular endothelium* lines the pulmonary circulation. The capillary endothelium constitutes approximately 50% of the cells in the lung parenchyma. As noted earlier, these cells have an intimate association with the type I pneumocyte. The vascular endothelium may have other regulatory functions in controlling vascular smooth muscle tone.

Fibroblasts. These are the cells of the interstitium (along with inflammatory cells, neural elements, and other cells). Lung fibroblasts synthesize and secrete *collagen* and *elastin*. These structural extracellular proteins determine the physiological characteristics of lung function. The collagenous skeleton of the lung forms the structural characteristics that ultimately limit lung distensibility. Elastin is a protein that, by virtue of its structural conformation, contributes to lung elastic recoil.

Connective tissue components are evident early in gestation (i.e., by the fourth week). Some fibroblasts (myofibroblasts) also have contractile properties. The proliferation of fibroblasts that synthesize collagen in pathological states during childhood or adulthood is the major cause of restrictive lung disease. The etiologies of these pathological proliferative states are numerous and varied.

Cartilage. The conducting airways of the lung are supported largely by cartilage, which progresses from the ringed formation of the trachea to the circumferential cartilaginous plates of the bronchi. Cartilage is evident in the trachea and main bronchi by the seventh week after conception, and the process extends to more peripheral airways up to the 25th week.

Cartilage develops from aggregation of mesenchymal cells. As they grow and differentiate, extracellular matrix and tropocollagen are secreted. This results in the isolation of cells into lacunae and the evolution of mature chondrocytes. The relationship of cartilaginous plates in airways to smooth muscle bronchoconstriction is discussed in Chapter 12.

Cells Derived from Ectoderm

Cells derived from ectoderm predominantly make up the neural elements of the lung. Neural ganglia in the lung develop early in fetal life (by week 7). Airways develop at least four distinct types of motor innervation: (1) sympathetic innervation (derived from thoracic sympathetic ganglia; there also are indirect sympathetic effects on airways caused by circulating epinephrine secreted into the systemic circulation by the adrenal gland); (2) parasympathetic innervation from the branches of the vagus nerve; (3) nonadrenergic inhibitory innervation, which follows anatomical pathways with the vagus nerve; and (4) nonadrenergic noncholinergic stimulatory innervation (caused by antidromal C-fibers that secrete neurokinins). The functional details of these distinct innervations are outlined in Chapter 12.

Chapter 11

Lung Defenses

Minute ventilation in an adult human ranges from 6 to 8 liters/min at rest to more than 100 liters/min in strenuous exercise. A normal individual typically will breathe between 10,000 and 30,000 liters of air over a 24-hour period. In addition to the oxygen, nitrogen, argon, carbon dioxide, and other gases normally present in the atmosphere, inhaled air contains nitrogen oxides, sulfur oxides, carbon monoxide, ozone, volatile organic compounds, hydrocarbons, and other toxic gases. Ambient air also contains particulate material including pollen, ash, mineral dust, mold spores, organic particles, and numerous other substances. A major nonrespiratory requirement for the lung and airways involves the processing of inhaled particulate material for excretion and the repair or replacement of cells injured or affected by inhalation of toxic substances. To prevent infection, the lungs must also clear the airways of inhaled infectious particles, including spores, bacteria, and viruses.

AIRWAY CLEARANCE MECHANISMS

Since new particles and toxic substances are continually being inhaled, the clearance of material and repair of cells are continuous processes. The lungs have the ability to augment their capacity to clear inhaled material, and individuals who regularly inhale large loads of foreign material or who smoke usually have chronically stimulated clearance mechanisms. In today's urban industrial environments, the air quality is often much poorer than in rural locations. Hence, the inhaled load of foreign materials presents a greater burden on the clearance mechanisms of the respiratory system for individuals living in cities. Likewise, occupations in which airborne materials are inhaled present an increased challenge to the clearance mechanisms of the lung. By virtue of their higher toxicity or greater resistance to clearance, certain substances are especially likely

149

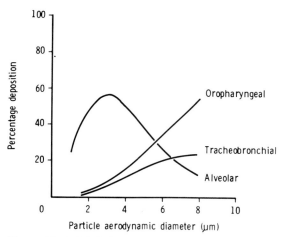

Figure 11–1. Inhaled particles tend to be trapped at different locations in the airways, depending on their size. Particles whose diameters are greater than about 5 μm tend to impact into the nasopharynx, oropharynx, or large conducting airways. Smaller particles are more likely to become trapped in the distal airways or in the alveoli. (From Clarke SW, Pavia D: Mucociliary clearance. In Crystal RG, West JB [eds]: The Lung: Scientific Foundation. New York, Raven Press, 1991, p 1846.)

to cause lung injury. Living or working in environments where excessive loads of foreign materials are inhaled can lead to the development of chronic lung injury, which often develops slowly over years or decades. Since early detection of this form of lung injury is difficult, diagnosis of occupation-induced lung disease frequently occurs only after significant lung disease has developed.

Deposition of Inhaled Particulate Material

Particulate material can be inhaled when it is stirred up into the air to form an *aerosol*. Aerosols are classified according to the size of the particles that they contain. An aerosol of large particles will tend to settle rapidly down to the floor in a sealed room, whereas an aerosol made of very fine particles will remain airborne for a much longer time. When airborne particles are inhaled, some of them become trapped as they contact the moist epithelial surface that lines the conducting airways or alveoli. The site where particles become trapped depends on the size of the particles, the mode of breathing (nose vs. mouth), the pattern of ventilation (tidal volume and frequency), and the size and shape of the airways.

Figure 11–1 shows the location where particles tend to become trapped, as a function of their diameter. Most particles with a diameter greater than about 5 μm tend to be trapped in the nasopharynx or oropharynx. By contrast, particles with diameters of less than 1 μm tend to become trapped in the tracheobronchial tree or in the distal airways and alveoli. Particles smaller than 1 μm have little chance of being trapped in the nasopharynx or conducting airways; most of these tend to become trapped in the distal lung regions or are exhaled.

Mechanisms of Particle Entrapment

Particles tend to become trapped in the epithelial surface for a variety of reasons. At points where the air stream changes direction (e.g., branch points), larger particles tend to *impact* into the surface because their inertia prevents them from changing direction rapidly. This is the primary mechanism of entrapment in the nasopharynx, where airflow velocities are high and the anatomical structures cause the flow to change direction rapidly. Turbulent flow regimens in the nasopharynx, trachea, and major bronchi also tend to enhance the impact of particles into the surface, because of eddies that travel perpendicular to the direction of flow. In more distal airways of the lung where flow velocities are lower, some particles settle out on the surface as a consequence of *gravitational* pull on them. Very small particles can contact the epithelium as they *diffuse* through alveolar gas.

Clearance of Entrapped Particulate Matter from the Conducting Airways

The cells that line the nasopharynx and conducting airways are ciliated, pseudostratified columnar epithelium. Mucous glands below the epithelium secrete mucus onto the epithelial surface that protects the epithelium and aids in clearance of trapped particles (Chapter 12). Within the epithelium are goblet cells that also secrete a viscous mucus onto the airway surface. The layer of mucus that blankets the airway surface is continuously moved by the cilia on the apical surface of the epithelial cells. Cilia in the nasopharynx beat in the direction to propel mucus down to the pharynx, while cilia in the trachea tend to propel mucus upward toward the pharynx, where it is swallowed. It is estimated that there are about 200 cilia per cell that beat at about 17 strokes per second. The mucous layer consists of a thick, viscous outer layer that glides over a thin, less viscous periciliary layer. The periciliary fluid provides a low-friction medium for the rapid movement of the cilia. During their active stroke, the tips of the cilia extend upward into the viscous layer, dragging it and the entrapped particles toward the pharynx. For this *mucociliary escalator* to function properly, the mucous layers must be of the proper thickness and viscosity. Mucus that is excessively thick or viscous cannot be moved effectively and may accumulate and obstruct the airway. Excessive mucus production can stress the ability of this clearance mechanism to keep the airways clear. Factors that interfere with ciliary motion or the density of cilia present in the airway can also inhibit clearance of mucus. Excess accumulation of mucus in the airways can stimulate the cough reflex, which helps to remove secretions. When functioning normally, the mucociliary clearance mechanism is highly effective and can normally clear particulate material deposited in the airways within a period of minutes to hours.

In moving from the conducting airways toward the alveoli there is a progressive change in the types of epithelial cells that are seen (Chapter 12). Unlike the ciliated columnar epithelium found in the conducting airways, alveoli are lined with nonciliated squamous epithelium. While goblet cells and submucosal glands are common along the conducting airways, they are not present in the alveoli. In traveling from the conducting airways toward the alveoli, the transition from ciliated to nonciliated epithelium is most noticeable beyond the terminal bronchioles. This transition also signals a change in the mechanism responsible for particle clearance, from mucociliary clearance (in the conducting airways) to the alveolar macrophage (within the alveoli and interstitial space). The transition region between ciliated airways and alveoli may also be the weakest in terms of clearance effectiveness. In patients with occupational lung diseases such as *pneumoconiosis* ("black lung disease" of coal miners), the highest concentration of particles is usually seen beyond the terminal bronchioles. It is likely that the relatively slow rate of clearance of particles at these sites provides an opportunity for the material to leave the airway and enter the interstitial space, where its clearance is extremely slow. Interestingly, this is frequently the primary site of airway damage in occupational lung diseases.

Clearance of Material from the Alveolar Space

Particles that are deposited on the alveolar walls or in alveolar ducts must be cleared by alveolar macrophages. Alveolar macrophages are large, mobile phagocytic cells that migrate through the alveoli and engulf foreign or effete autologous material. Most of these macrophages are found in the alveoli, although some can be found in the interstitium and a few others may be found wandering in the terminal airways. Lung macrophages are mononuclear cells derived from blood monocytes, which in turn are derived from bone marrow. Normally, most of the macrophages present in the lung are the result of secondary cell division by other alveolar macrophages. However, in states of chronic inflammation (e.g., tuberculosis) blood monocytes migrate into the lung and differentiate into new alveolar macrophages. This greatly increases the number of alveolar macrophages that can participate in fighting the infectious process.

Alveolar macrophages phagocytize foreign material as well as dead cells or cell debris. For phagocytosis to occur, both calcium and magnesium ions must be present in the environment. Some material that is phagocytosed is dissolved by the macrophage, while other material is merely engulfed. Macrophages have potent bactericidal, fungicidal, and virus killing abilities. Normally, the macrophage must engulf a potentially infectious organism to kill it. After it phagocytizes an infectious agent, it undergoes a burst in metabolic activity. The infectious organism is killed by oxygen radicals (e.g., hydrogen peroxide) or halogen derivatives (e.g., hypochlorous acid) synthesized by the macrophage. In addition to their role in clearing particulate material from the alveolar space, these macrophages also play an active role in the immune response through their interactions with lymphocytes. They also participate in cell-mediated immunity and in the detection and destruction of neoplastic cells within the lung.

Alveolar macrophages clear unwanted material from the alveolar space rapidly. If a load of inhaled particles is deposited in the alveoli, alveolar macrophages will phagocytize about 25% of them within 1 hour. By 24 hours, the entire load will have been phagocytosed. After ingesting a load of particles, the macrophage may remain within the alveolar space or may leave the lung through several different routes. Some migrate into the airways where they can be transported up to the pharynx in the mucociliary escalator. Others appear to exit from the lung by entering the lymphatic system. Still others may die within the alveolar space, where their remains are cleared by other alveolar macrophages.

In general, the longer the inhaled material remains in the lung, the greater the probability that lung damage will occur. By clearing material rapidly, alveolar macrophages prevent particles from escaping from the alveoli into the interstitial space of the lung. When particles do enter the interstitium, they are cleared much more slowly and are therefore more likely to induce tissue injury.

PATHOPHYSIOLOGY OF ALVEOLAR MACROPHAGES

Although the alveolar macrophage plays an important role in defending the lung against injury or infection under normal circumstances, there are situations in which the macrophage may contribute to lung injury. For example, if toxic or radioactive particles are accidentally inhaled into the lung, the phagocytosis of the particles by macrophages tends to concentrate the material into small regions of the lung. The higher concentration of toxic material in these "hot spots" may increase the local tissue injury.

Phagocytosis of toxic materials can cause injury or death to the macrophage. Materials can be toxic to the macrophage because of chemical toxicity or because the material is not readily digested by the cell. For example, silica dust or asbestos fibers are mineral crystals that cannot be dissolved after phagocytosis. These sharp crystals can tear through lysosomes within the macrophage that ingests them, resulting in its death. Chemotactic factors released from dead or dying macrophages cause fibroblasts to migrate into the region and stimulate them to synthesize new collagen. As new macrophages migrate into the region and ingest the dead macrophages, they, too, are killed by the debris. Their death stimulates the migration of additional fibroblasts and the synthesis of more collagen. This

process can develop into a vicious cycle and cause the accumulation of excess collagen in the lung. This can lead to the development of *pulmonary interstitial fibrosis*, a disease associated with reduced lung compliance, impaired gas exchange, and an increased work of breathing.

Increased numbers of alveolar macrophages and polymorphonuclear leukocytes (neutrophils) are typically found in the lungs of individuals who smoke or who otherwise inhale large quantities of aerosolized particles. When a macrophage encounters foreign particles in the lung, it is transformed into an activated state. This activation is associated with an increased cellular metabolic rate and an increased rate of phagocytosis. Activated macrophages and neutrophils tend to release small quantities of elastase enzymes during phagocytosis, which are capable of degrading extracellular structural proteins such as elastin. In normal lungs, other enzymes called *antiproteases* inactivate these proteases, thereby limiting their tissue destruction. However, the balance between the ability of the lung to inactivate these enzymes and their rate of release can be disrupted in individuals who chronically inhale large loads of particles. When unopposed protease activity continues unchecked, a state of chronic inflammation can develop that leads to the degradation of alveolar septal walls that can progress to *emphysema*. Some individuals with congenital α_1-antitrypsin deficiency lack the ability to synthesize this important antiprotease enzyme. This deficiency predisposes these persons to the development of emphysema at an early age (30–40 years old). Studies indicate that these individuals develop emphysema even earlier if they smoke or work unprotected in dusty environments.

Hyperoxic Lung Injury

Molecular oxygen is required for normal cell metabolic activity, but it can be toxic to cells if they are exposed to high concentrations. When patients with acute lung gas exchange failure are given high oxygen concentrations to breathe, the cells of the lung and airways may sustain injury from the high oxygen concentration in a condition known as *oxygen toxicity*. The likelihood of encountering oxygen toxicity varies with the concentration of oxygen used and the duration of exposure. For example, among humans ventilated with 100% oxygen, about half

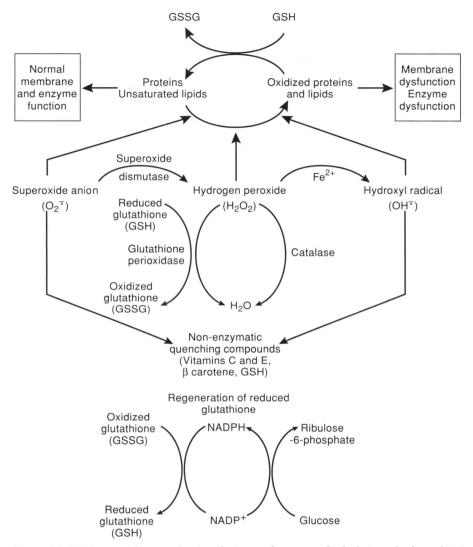

Figure 11–2. Schematic diagram showing the types of oxygen radicals that can be formed in hyperoxic lung injury, the sites of cell damage, and the mechanisms available for their inactivation. (GSH: reduced glutathione; GSSG: oxidized glutathione) See text for further explanation.

will show signs of oxygen toxicity after 4 to 7 days. However, if less than 60% oxygen is used, the likelihood of developing signs of oxygen toxicity is much lower. Although many cells of the body are susceptible to hyperoxic injury, the cells of the lung are usually the first to manifest the effects of oxygen toxicity since they are the ones exposed to the highest concentrations.

Experimental evidence suggests that the tissue injury associated with oxygen toxicity is caused by

the production of toxic free radicals, which can be formed both intracellularly and extracellularly. The rate of oxygen radical production increases at higher levels of tissue P_{O_2}. This explains why hyperoxic lung injury tends to be worse when higher concentrations of oxygen are inhaled. Cell damage occurs when free radicals react actively with lipids, proteins, or deoxyribonucleic acid (DNA), leading to a disruption of cell membranes, interference with intracellular processes, or disruption of membrane transport. When a free radical reacts with a molecule, the molecule itself becomes a highly reactive radical capable of reacting with and altering other nearby molecules. Consequently, the generation of oxygen free radicals can initiate a chain reaction of radical generation and molecular damage. When the cumulative tissue damage becomes severe, evidence of impaired organ function becomes evident.

Figure 11–2 summarizes the various types of oxygen radicals and the mechanisms that contribute to tissue injury. Evidence suggests that different oxygen radicals can damage cells by different mechanisms. *Superoxide anion* (O_2^-) is formed within mitochondria when only one electron is transferred to molecular oxygen. Some superoxide ions are generated in mitochondria at normal oxygen tensions, but their rate of production is greatly enhanced at high oxygen concentrations. Superoxide anions selectively damage certain enzymes and can also attack unsaturated fatty acids, causing lipid peroxidation. *Superoxide dismutase* converts superoxide anions into *hydrogen peroxide,* which can easily enter cells by diffusing through the cell membrane. Hydrogen peroxide damages cells by causing strand breaks in nuclear DNA. In the presence of ferrous iron ions (Fe^{2+}), the *hydroxyl radical* can be formed from hydrogen peroxide. Hydroxyl radicals are extremely toxic and react immediately with any nearby molecules. Hydroxyl radicals can contribute to lipid peroxidation, DNA damage, and protein damage.

Oxygen toxicity in the lung is manifested by damage to alveolar type I cells, pulmonary endothelial cells, and alveolar macrophages. Although alveolar type II cells are also susceptible to oxygen toxicity, they appear less sensitive than the other cell types and often proliferate in response to hyperoxia. Experimental studies indicate that initial hyperoxic damage to endothelial and alveolar type I cells leads to interstitial and alveolar edema formation. Cell division in the lung becomes inhibited, and an inflammatory process is initiated. Later in the injury process, lung fibroblasts proliferate and increase their production of collagen. This can lead to the development of pulmonary interstitial fibrosis when the injury is severe. The net effect of pulmonary oxygen toxicity reflects a balance between the rate at which tissue injury proceeds and the rate of tissue repair. If the rate of oxygen radical production and tissue injury does not greatly outweigh the ability of the lung to repair itself, then little functional impairment may be evident.

Several mechanisms are available to defend the lung against the effects of hyperoxic exposure. First, specific substances can *quench* the chain reaction of free radicals by scavenging them. Substances such as vitamin E, beta-carotene (a vitamin A precursor), and vitamin C are examples of effective free radical scavengers. Cells can *degrade* toxic oxygen radicals using three complementary intracellular antioxidant systems. Among these, *catalase* is an enzyme that catalyzes the degradation of hydrogen peroxide into water and molecular oxygen. *Superoxide dismutase* is an enzyme that converts superoxide anion into hydrogen peroxide, a less reactive molecule. Reduced *glutathione* contributes to the degradation of large molecule hydroperoxides and lipid peroxides. This is an important intracellular mechanism because reduced glutathione is present in relatively high concentrations in cells and oxidized glutathione can be recycled to reduced glutathione enzymatically. Under some circumstances, it is possible to *limit the production* of oxygen radicals by limiting the substrate or the stimulus for oxidant production. Finally, cells can proceed with the *tissue repair* process, even before the stimulus for oxidant production is removed.

Chapter 12

Biology of Conducting Airways

GROSS ANATOMY

The conducting airways of the lung refer to those airways that connect the outside world to the alveoli. These airways "deliver" and "excrete" the air to the alveoli, but they are not involved in gas exchange with blood. There is an enormous arborization of the conducting airways starting from the trachea, so that the cross-sectional area of the airways (a single 2- to 3-cm² diameter airway at the trachea) is massive at the alveolar level (greater than 10,000 cm²) in the adult lung. Figure 12–1 shows the gross divisions of lung from the trachea into *bronchopulmonary segments*. The right lung has three lobes (upper, middle, and lower), and the left lung has two lobes (upper and lower). There are 10 bronchopulmonary segments of the right lung and 9 of the left lung (note there is no segment 7 on the left). The left lung is smaller than the right because of the volume occupied by the heart.

The exact number of airway generations is not known. It has been estimated that there are 23 to 24 generations of airways (the trachea is classified as generation 0), but as many as 27 generations may exist (Figure 12–2). Figure 12–3 shows the tremendous increase in cross-sectional area of the airways that occurs, especially after the first 7 airway generations (note that the ordinate is the logarithm of the total cross-sectional area at each level of airway generation).

The Upper Airways

The nose is the first structure in series with the conducting airways, and it functions as an air-

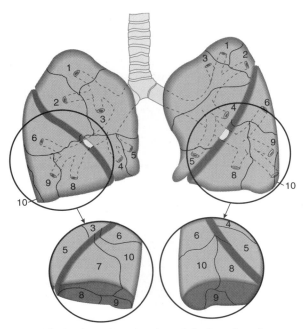

Figure 12–1. *Above:* Anterior view of the bronchopulmonary segments of the lung. A discrete middle lobe (segments 4 and 5 in the right lung) is replaced in the left lung by a lingula in the upper lobe providing space for the left ventricular prominence. *Below (encircled):* Posterior view of the numbered segments in lower lung fields.

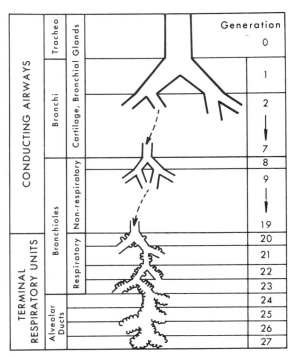

Figure 12–2. Branching of the conducting airways. There are between 23 and 27 generations of airways. (From Weibel ER: Morphometry of the Human Lung. Berlin, Springer-Verlag, 1963.)

conditioning and filtering device. The volume of the nose is approximately 20 ml, but it has an extensive mucosal surface consisting of the nasal *turbinates.* The nasal turbinates are the chambers of the nasal cavity through which air flows before reaching the *oropharynx.* The resistance to airflow through the nose is substantial (~ 8 cm H_2O/liter/sec) and may become very large during viral infections or with allergies (allergic rhinitis), prompting the subject to switch to "mouth breathing." The nose is the first in a series of temperature- and moisture-conditioning airways that warm and humidify the air. The mucous layer of the nose and the tortuous structure of the turbinates serve to filter particulates and prevent these from reaching more distal airways. This is the first stage of filtration. The flow of mucus clears the main nasal passages approximately every 15 minutes in normal individuals. Nasal secretions contain some important immunoglobulins, inflammatory cells, and interferon, which are the first step in host defenses against viruses. Some patients suffer from nasal polyps, which block the nasal pas-

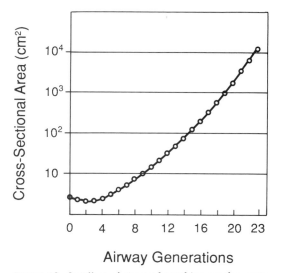

Figure 12–3. Effect of airway branching on the cross-sectional area of the lung. Note that the ordinate is a logarithmic scale. (From Weibel ER: Morphometry of the Human Lung. Berlin, Springer-Verlag, 1963.)

sages completely. These patients must become "mouth breathers" and may lose their sense of taste. Taste is dependent on olfaction, and closed nasal passages block access for the vapors of food and the perception of taste.

The larynx is the second structure in the line of conduction. Under certain conditions (e.g., vocal cord spasm or infection) it can become a source of considerable resistance to airflow. The larynx is also the organ for both speech and singing. The epiglottis covers the upper airway when subjects are not breathing and thus is a physical barrier for food and other substances contained in the mouth; this prevents aspiration into the lung.

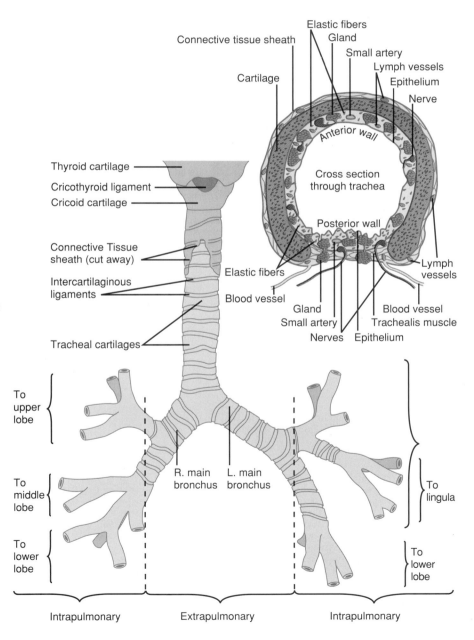

Figure 12–4. *Left:* Structure of the extrapulmonary airways. The cartilage surrounding the airway confers considerable rigidity in comparison with the more peripheral airways. For the trachea, the cartilage is arranged in a horseshoe pattern anteriorly, and all of the tracheal smooth muscle, neural supply, and vascular tissue originate from the posterior membrane (see cross section). The horseshoe arrangement of cartilage is preserved at the first branch into the mainstem bronchi; however, with subsequent branching, the cartilage becomes arranged circumferentially into discontinuous plates (see Figure 12–5). *Right:* Cross-section through the trachea, showing horseshoe distribution of cartilage at this level.

The upper airways also "condition" inspired air, and by the time inspired air reaches the distal airways it is humidified and warmed to body temperature.

The Trachea and Main Bronchi

The trachea is continuous with the upper airway and the larynx. It begins at the level of the seventh cervical vertebra and ends at the second thoracic vertebra where it divides at the *carina* into the *mainstem bronchi* to the right and left lungs. The anterior (ventral) portion of the trachea is somewhat rigid because it contains tracheal cartilages, which are horseshoe shaped and are arranged as shown in

Figure 12–4. These cartilaginous rings extend about 270 degrees to the posterior (dorsal) surface, and each cartilaginous ring (approximately 18 in total) is spanned by a *ligamentous membrane*. The posterior membrane of the trachea forms a flat surface that is lined by a continuation of the epithelial membrane. Beneath this epithelial surface lies the remainder of the posterior membrane, which consists of horizontally oriented tracheal smooth muscle that may pull the loop of the horseshoe cartilage together, thus making the airway even more rigid.

At the *carina*, the mainstem bronchi make an angle of about 85 degrees from the trachea. Beginning with generation 3, the subsequent divisions of airways are contained within the parenchyma of the lung (Figure 12–5). The attachment to the elastic tissue of the surrounding lung opposes airway collapse during forced expiration (see Chapter 2). Destruction of lung parenchymal tissue, as occurs in emphysema, causes loss of these tethering forces and thus promotes collapse during expiration.

The mainstem bronchi somewhat resemble the

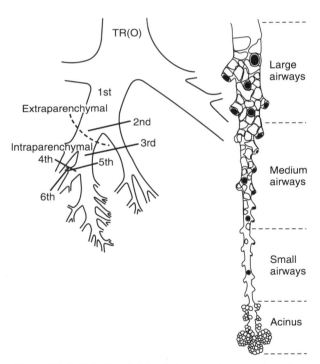

Figure 12–5. *Left.* The division between extraparenchymal airways and intraparenchymal airways. The latter are distended by lung matrix forces (see text). *Right.* Further branching of the parenchymal airways showing the discontinuous cartilaginous plates that are connected by airway smooth muscle in the bronchi. These merge by gradual transition into the bronchioles, the most distal of which (the respiratory bronchiole) are the terminal conducting airways leading to the alveolar ducts and alveoli, which are gas exchange units. (Left figure is redrawn from Shioya T, Munoz N, Leff AR: Translation of contractile force to constriction in major diameter canine airways in vivo. Am Rev Respir Dis 140:688, 1989.)

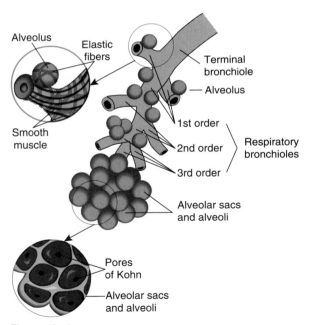

Figure 12–6. Transition of the terminal bronchiole to the gas exchange units of the lung. The alveoli are amuscular saccules having a rich vascular supply from the pulmonary circulation for gas exchange. *Circled above:* Detailed view of anatomical relationship. *Circled below:* Inside view of alveoli (luminal side) demonstrating interalveolar communications through the pores of Kohn.

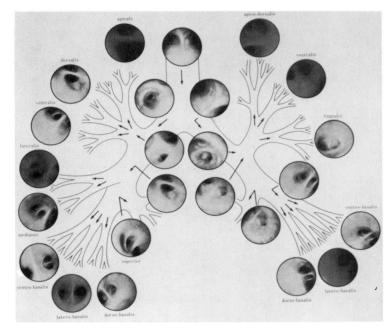

Figure 12–7. The conducting airways of the lung as viewed through the fiberoptic bronchoscope. (From Nagaishi C: Functional Anatomy and Histology of the Lung [American edition]. New York, Igaku-Shoin, 1972.)

trachea. Much of the cartilaginous tissue is anterior, and there is a posterior membrane similar to that of the trachea. However, as the bronchi branch progressively, the cartilaginous distribution becomes circumferential and discontinuous. Airway smooth muscle is helically wound around the entire airway (Figure 12–6). As arborization continues, the cartilaginous content of the bronchi diminishes and the airways progressively adopt the microscopic saccular arrangement of the alveoli (Figure 12–6). Figure 12–7 presents a view through the bronchoscope.

The large conducting airways are supplied by the bronchial circulation. This is a systemic circulation, part of which drains into the pulmonary circulation. From the hilum to the periphery, there is a dual blood supply to the airways from the bronchial (systemic) and pulmonary (right side of the heart–derived) circulations. The alveoli are supplied exclusively by the pulmonary capillaries.

HISTOLOGICAL ORGANIZATION

The conducting airways have three major components of their wall: (1) a luminal mucosa that is composed of epithelium and lamina propria (the latter is absent in the gas exchange airways); (2) airway smooth muscle; and (3) in larger airways, a submucosal connective layer, which also contains the blood supply to the airway. In larger airways, blood vessels also course through the lamina propria. In the conducting airways of the lung, the epithelial layer contains ciliated pseudostratified columnar epithelial cells. The cilia cells propel mucus from the distal to the proximal airways (see Chapter 10). This epithelium is substantially thicker than the very thin epithelial cells of the alveoli (Figure 12–8). Figure 12–9 is a photomicrograph showing the epithelium of large and small airways.

The smooth muscle layer of the conducting airways is oriented to facilitate airway narrowing. As noted, this orientation is transverse in the trachea, and contraction narrows the horseshoe portion of the cartilage. Because of the substantial elasticity of the tracheal cartilage and the limited area in which there is a muscle, tracheal constriction is limited. In more distal conducting airways, the geometric pattern of smooth muscle orientation, which is wrapped entirely around the airway, allows for more complete narrowing. However, the narrowing of parenchymal airways is opposed by the lung tissue that tethers these airways open (see earlier).

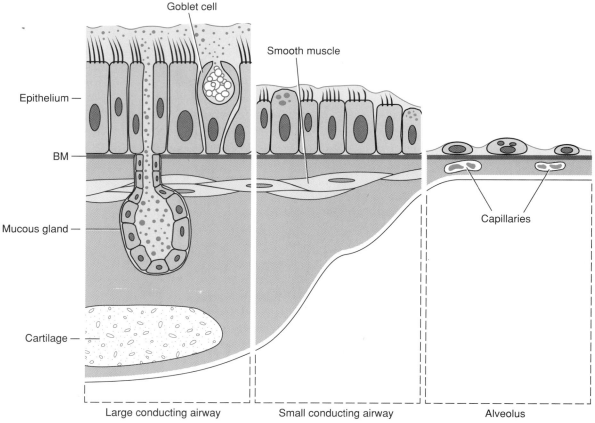

Figure 12-8. Transition from the large conducting airways of the lung to the gas exchange units: schema. The basic organization remains the same. However, the epithelium, which serves a major barrier function in the upper airways, thins to become a more permeable membrane in close continuity with a rich vascular bed in the alveoli. Gradually, the cartilage and, finally, the airway smooth muscle are lost so that the alveoli are an efficient membrane exchange system.

Figure 12-10 shows the histological relationships between epithelium and airway muscle in cross-sections from a conducting airway.

As demonstrated in Figure 12-8, the relative composition of the major components of the conducting airways undergoes a gradual transition. In the distal peripheral airways, ciliation is lost and mucous glands and cartilage are no longer present. Airway smooth muscle exists, however, down to alveolar duct level. A large but extremely thin membrane surface remains at the alveolar level. Cells of the alveoli secrete surfactant (alveolar type II cells), but mucus is not secreted in the alveoli or in the most distal airways (Figure 12-11).

Other Cellular Constituents of Conducting Airways

Fluid obtained from *alveolar lavage* (rinse) contains large numbers of alveolar macrophages. In patients with inflammatory conditions of the lung, white blood cell granulocytes (eosinophils, neutrophils) migrate into the airways. In asthma, eosinophils are often a predominant infiltrate of the conducting airways (Figure 12-12). In bacterial pneumonia, polymorphonuclear leukocytes infiltrate the alveolar spaces and phagocytize bacterial pathogens (Figure 12-13).

Mast cells are derived from basophils and share

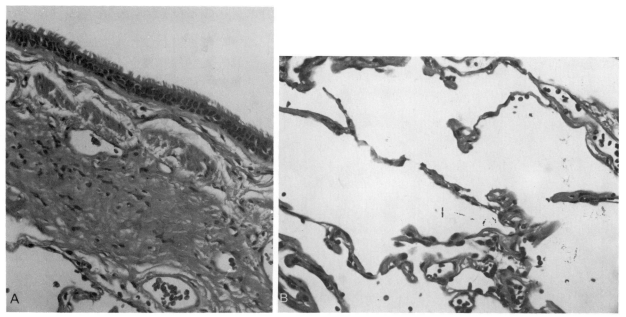

Figure 12-9. The epithelium of a bronchus *(A)* and the alveolus *(B)*. Note the ciliated arrangement in the conducting airways, which also contain numerous goblet cells. The alveolus has an extremely thin epithelium. Its secretory cells are the type II cells (see Figure 12-12), which synthesize and secrete surfactant. (Photomicrographs courtesy of Dr. Cyril Abrahams, University of Chicago.)

Figure 12-10. Histology of the conducting airways. In the bronchus (generation 4 or 5) the cartilage is arranged circumferentially about the airways. Contraction of smooth muscle tethered between the cartilaginous plates constricts the airway. (Photomicrograph courtesy of Dr. Cyril Abrahams, University of Chicago.)

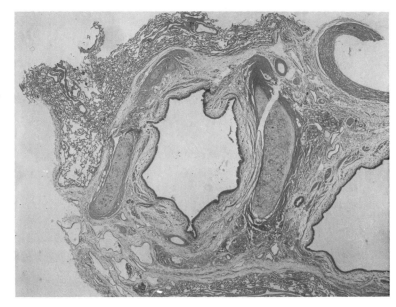

osmiophilic lamellar bodies

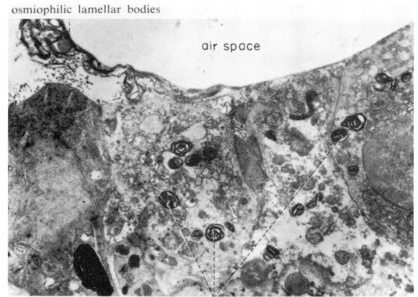

air space

osmiophilic lamellar bodies

Figure 12–11. The cellular population of the alveoli stained histologically to demonstrate alveolar type II cells. Note osmophilic (electron dense) lamellar bodies for surfactant secretion. (From Nagaishi C: Functional Anatomy and Histology of the Lung. Baltimore, University Park Press, 1971, p. 51.)

many of the properties of their precursors. They are rich in histamine and capable of synthesizing a large variety of mediators that cause airway mucosal edema and smooth muscle contraction in conducting airways. These mediators include various prostaglandins (e.g., prostaglandins D_2 and $F_{2\alpha}$, thromboxane A_2, leukotrienes, and platelet activating factor). Mast cells reside on the luminal epithelial surface and also within the airway wall in proximity to airway smooth muscle (Figure 12–14). Mast cells release preformed mediators from cytoplasmic granules when activated. One mechanism by which mast cells are activated is through immune sensitization in certain *atopic* (allergic) individuals. Inha-

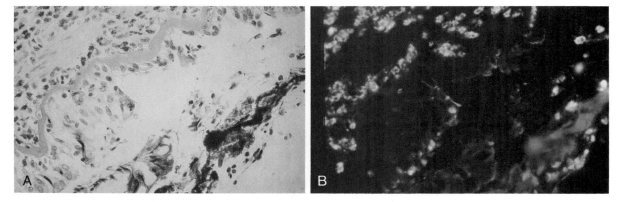

Figure 12–12. Infiltration of eosinophils into the conducting airways in asthma. These are the predominant granulocytic constituent of these airways. *A.* Hematoxylin and eosin stain. *B.* Immune fluorescent stain for eosinophils. (From Gleich GJ, et al: The eosinophil as a mediator of damage to respiratory epithelium: A model for bronchial hyperactivity. J Allergy Clin Immunol 81:776–781, 1988. Photomicrographs [×450] courtesy of Dr. Gerald Gleich, Mayo Foundation, Rochester, MN.)

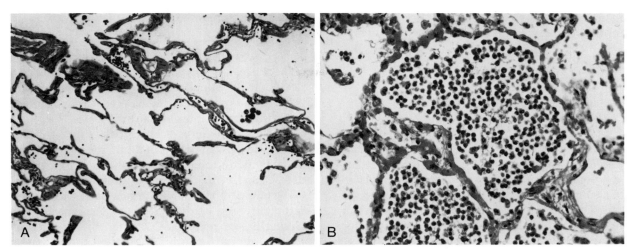

Figure 12-13. Infiltration of polymorphonuclear leukocytes into the alveolar space with acute bacterial pneumonia. Compare infected lung *(B)* with the normal histology *(A)*. (Photomicrographs [×450] courtesy of Dr. Cyril Abrahams, University of Chicago.)

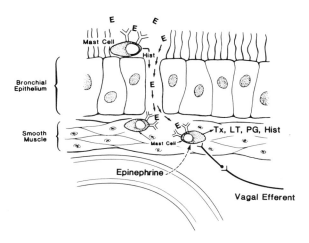

Figure 12-14. Activation of respiratory mast cells by antigen E. Bivalent linkage of IgE antibodies with specific antigens causes active secretion of mediators at the surface, including histamine (Hist). This opens the tight junctions of the conducting airways, which normally are highly impermeable, and allows delivery of antigen to the deeper layers of the airway. Here mast cells interspersed within airway smooth muscle are activated; this causes both bronchoconstriction and edema from fluid leakage from the bronchial blood vessels. Tx, thromboxane; LT, leukotrienes; PG, prostaglandins; E, antigen E. (From Leff A: State of the art: Endogenous regulation of bronchomotor tone. Am Rev Respir Dis 137:1198–1216, 1988.)

lation of antigens, such as ragweed pollen or cat dander, causes synthesis of immunoglobulin E (IgE) by plasma cells. This antigen-specific IgE then binds to mast cells, causing activation of the mast cell (see Figure 12-14) and release of mediators locally into the tissues of the nose and airways. In some individuals (about 40 million in the United States), this is the mechanism of *allergic rhinitis* (e.g., hay fever). In others, the release of mediators into bronchial airways causes airway edema and narrowing (i.e., *asthma*).

Figure 12-14 demonstrates the presumed mechanism by which mast cell activation by IgE antigen–antibody complexing causes bronchoconstriction in susceptible individuals. Binding of antigen E to IgE on mast cells at the epithelial surface opens the tight junctions of the epithelium, which normally serves as a barrier. This is caused by the release of histamine from activated respiratory mast cells, and it allows further penetration of specific antigen E to the deeper respiratory mast cells that are immediately adjacent to the airway smooth muscle. Bronchoactive and edemagenic mediators (promoting vascular leakage into the tissues) are released. When individuals have allergic rhinitis, the nasal mucosa becomes swollen. The same phenomenon causes itching of the nose and eye. When the individual is also susceptible to asthma, the process causes contraction of airway smooth muscle and constriction of the conducting airways.

NEUROHUMORAL REGULATION OF CONDUCTING AIRWAYS

Innervation of the airways is entirely autonomic. There is no voluntary motor innervation to the airways nor are there any pain fibers in airways. (There are also no pain fibers in the lung parenchyma, but there is considerable innervation with pain fibers in the pleura.) There are both visceral sensory (afferent) and visceral motor (efferent) nerves that affect airway function.

Afferent and Reflex-Mediated Responses in Airways

Slowly Adapting Receptors. These receptors are named because the rate of firing accommodates slowly to a stimulus. Parasympathetic output through the vagus nerve is the predominant source of resting smooth muscle tone in airways. The reflex caused by stimulation of slowly adapting receptors in the airway wall results in inhibition of parasympathetic motor tone that occurs with each inspiration. Deep inspiration, which inhibits parasympathetic output, also inhibits bronchomotor tone. The receptor for the "stretch" reflex, which is part of the Hering-Breuer reflex (see Chapter 8), is located in the periphery of the lung (Figure 12–15) and is associated with the lung parenchyma. Dilation of

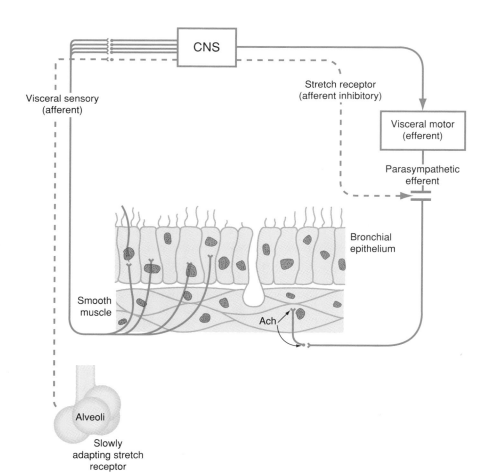

Figure 12–15. Component of Hering-Breuer reflex in the lung. Slowly adapting stretch receptors (visceral afferent) transmit an impulse to the central nervous system, which causes preganglionic inhibition of vagal tone to airway smooth muscle. The result is that airway smooth muscle relaxes with an inspiration. (From Leff A: State of the art: Endogenous regulation of bronchomotor tone. Am Rev Respir Dis 137:1198–1216, 1988.)

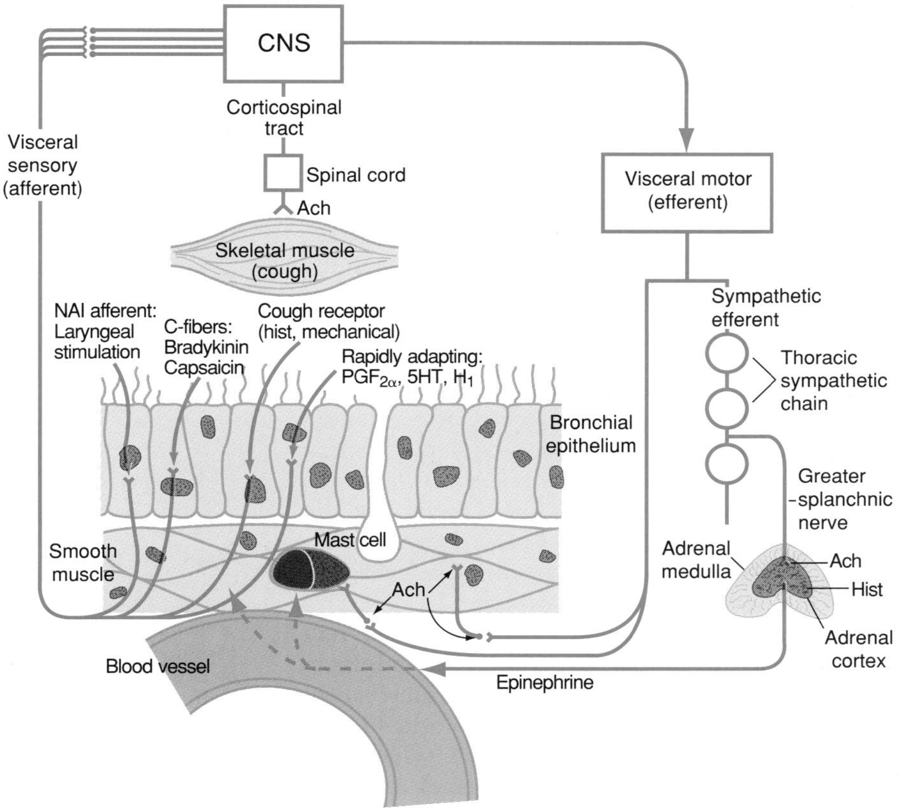

Figure 12-16. Other sensorimotor reflexes in the lung. Receptors located in the epithelium transmit afferent stimuli through the vagus nerve to the central nervous system (CNS). These are translated into a variety of efferent stimuli including cough, bronchodilation, and bronchoconstriction (see text for details). NAI, nonadrenergic, noncholinergic inhibitory; hist, histamine; PGF$_{2\alpha}$, prostaglandin F$_{2\alpha}$; 5HT, serotonin; H$_1$, H$_1$ histamine receptor; Ach, acetylcholine. (From Leff A: State of the art: Endogenous regulation of bronchomotor tone. Am Rev Respir Dis 137:1198-1216, 1988.)

CNS

Corticospinal tract

Visceral sensory (afferent)

Spinal cord

Ach

Skeletal muscle (cough)

Visceral motor (efferent)

Sympathetic efferent

Thoracic sympathetic chain

Greater -splanchnic nerve

NAI afferent: Laryngeal stimulation

C-fibers: Bradykinin Capsaicin

Cough receptor (hist, mechanical)

Rapidly adapting: PGF$_{2\alpha}$, 5HT, H$_1$

Bronchial epithelium

Smooth muscle

Mast cell

Ach

Adrenal medulla

Ach

Hist

Adrenal cortex

Blood vessel

Epinephrine

Figure 12-17. Parasympathetic mediation of reflex bronchoconstriction: schematic representation of experiments. Unilateral administration of antigen (right lung) causes bilateral narrowing of airways. Right vagotomy blocks the response on both sides, demonstrating the reflex nature of the efferent response. (From Leff AR: Toward the formation of a modern theory of asthma. Perspect Biol Med 33:292-302, 1990. Reproduced by permission of the University of Chicago Press.)

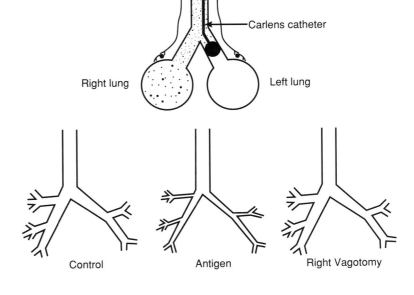

Vagus nerve

Vagus nerve

Carlens catheter

Right lung

Left lung

Control

Antigen

Right Vagotomy

the proximal conducting airways has no effect on parasympathetic tone, although this may elicit stress-relaxation of the smooth muscle itself.

Rapidly Adapting Receptors. These sensory fibers reside in the epithelium of the large airways. The name is derived from their physiological characteristic of adapting rapidly to a stimulus. When the stimulus is initiated, these sensory fibers fire rapidly and then quickly accommodate to slow firing of neural impulses. Rapidly adapting receptors are also called *irritant receptors* because irritation and inflammation (including mediators released during immune activation, e.g., histamine, prostaglandin $F_{2\alpha}$) stimulate firing of these nerves. Stimulation of the irritant receptor initiates a reflex that results in bronchoconstriction. Irritant fibers travel through the vagus nerve to the central nervous system. Efferent parasympathetic signals travel back through the vagus nerve to the airways (Figure 12–16). This causes bronchoconstriction by increasing efferent parasympathetic output. Experimental administration of antigen (Figure 12–17) to one lung causes bilateral bronchoconstriction that is blocked (1) by cooling the afferent vagus on the side to which antigen is administered (afferent blockage) or (2) by giving atropine (efferent blockade) or performing right vagotomy. Patients with asthma have a hyperreactive irritant receptor response, as do normal subjects who develop viral infections of the upper airways (Figure 12–18).

Cough Reflex. The cough reflex links an afferent visceral sensory stimulus to activation of an efferent somatic motor response. The afferent receptor is a component of the autonomic nervous system. The efferent component of the cough reflex is the forceful movement of skeletal muscle to effect the cough. Although the mechanism is not understood completely, the cough threshold is lowered by stimuli that cause bronchoconstriction. Patients with asthma have increased cough, and this is diminished by treatment that causes bronchodilation.

Cold and Exercise: C-Fibers. Many individuals develop mild bronchoconstriction following cold air *hyperpnea* (increased ventilation). This response is more pronounced in individuals with asthma. The mechanism by which cold air causes bronchoconstriction is not fully understood. However, respira-

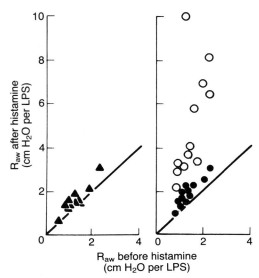

Figure 12–18. Effect of inhalation of histamine on airway resistance (R_{aw}) in normal human subjects with respiratory viral infections (common colds). Data are plotted against lines of identity. *Left.* Individuals not having viral infection. Histamine causes only slight bronchoconstriction as indicated by close fit to the line of identity. *Right.* Normal individuals with upper respiratory viral infections (colds). Histamine causes a major increase in R_{aw} *(open circles)*, which returns to control state after recovery from cold *(solid circles)*. The hyperresponsiveness *(open circles)* is blocked by atropine, which blocks parasympathetic transmission. (From Empey DW, et al: Mechanisms of bronchial hyperreactivity in normal subjects after upper respiratory tract infection. Am Rev Respir Dis 113:131–139, 1976.)

tory *heat loss* and *water loss* have been shown to correlate with the bronchoconstriction in subjects with exercise-induced bronchoconstriction. Neither the afferent nor the efferent limb of this response is defined fully. Currently, it is believed that C-fibers in the airways may be involved in this response. Release of *tachykinins* (such as the peptides *substance P* and *neurokinin A*) from C-fibers may mediate the bronchoconstrictive response to cold air hyperpnea. These neurokinins initiate both vascular leakage of fluid into the airway (edema) and direct bronchoconstriction of airway smooth muscle. Neurokinins are metabolized endogenously at the surface of the epithelium by the enzyme neutral endopeptidase. Inhibition of this enzyme greatly augments the activity of neurokinin-mediated responses. In experimental animal models (Figure 12–19), hyperventilation has been shown to cause bronchoconstriction and edema, which are

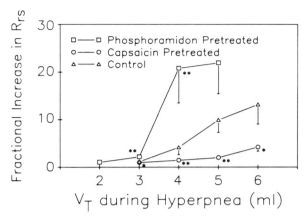

Figure 12–19. Nonadrenergic noncholinergic stimulatory (NANC) nerves: effect of respiratory cooling/ hyperventilation on respiratory system resistance (R_{rs}) in a guinea pig. With increase in tidal volume (Vt), an increase in minute ventilation is elicited; there is a concomitant increase in R_{rs} to 13 times the baseline value *(triangles)*. When animals are pretreated with an agent that ablates the NANC nerves (C-fibers) in the airways, the response to hyperventilation is blunted substantially *(circles)*. The airway smooth muscle contractile response causing the increase in R_{rs} is thought to be caused by neurokinins. Pretreatment with phosphoramidon, an inhibitor of the neutral endopeptidase enzyme that degrades neurokinins, greatly augments the response to hyperventilation *(squares)*. (From Ray DW, et al: Tachykinins mediate bronchoconstriction elicited by isocapnic hyperpnea in guinea pigs. J Appl Physiol 66:1108–1112, 1989.)

(1) augmented by blockade of neutral endopeptidase enzyme and (2) prevented by obliteration of C-fibers.

Dyspnea. Dyspnea is the perception of shortness of breath (i.e., it is a symptom). As it relates to the conducting airways, dyspnea results from the increased work of breathing that occurs when airways narrow. Patients with acute asthma have severe dyspnea, which often causes them to hyperventilate to a $Paco_2$ substantially below the normal level of 40 torr. In fact, a "normal" $Paco_2$ in severe asthma is considered an ominous sign because dyspnea is such a powerful stimulus during severe airway narrowing that the failure to demonstrate a decreased Pco_2 implies respiratory muscle fatigue and imminent respiratory arrest. The power of this stimulus is indicated by the propensity of patients with severe airway narrowing to use their respiratory muscles to the point of fatigue.

EFFERENT RESPONSES IN CONDUCTING AIRWAYS

The airways are innervated by four separate components of the autonomic nervous system: (1) the parasympathetic nervous system; (2) the sympathetic nervous system; (3) the nonadrenergic, noncholinergic (NANC) nervous inhibitory system; and (4) NANC-stimulatory nerves (C-fibers). [The C-fibers discussed earlier are currently classified as one component of the NANC system.]

Parasympathetic Innervation

The airways are innervated by the parasympathetic nervous system. Tonic parasympathetic activity maintains a mild but continuous degree of airway smooth muscle contraction (tone). Parasympathetic innervation is most significant in the major airways of the lung and diminishes toward the periphery, terminating in the small conducting airways. Parasympathetic nerves also innervate the mucous glands of the airways, and their stimulation is associated with the increased mucus production that occurs during respiratory tract infections or irritation. Mucous glands are also innervated by sympathetic nerves. Parasympathetic stimulation increases production of mucus glycoproteins, while sympathetic stimulation causes a more watery secretion. Thus, the viscosity of mucus secretion is a function, at least in part, of autonomic balance between these systems. The role of reflex parasympathetic stimulation on bronchomotor tone has been discussed earlier.

The anatomy of the parasympathetic nervous system permits discrete efferent regulation of visceral function. A long preganglionic fiber courses from the nucleus of the XI cranial nerve through the vagus nerve to discrete ganglia, located in the adventitia of the tissue that it innervates (Figure 12–20). This permits parasympathetic control of a single organ. For example, changes in bronchomotor tone may occur independently of changes in gut peristalsis.

Sympathetic Innervation

In contrast to the organization of the parasympathetic nervous system, activation of the sympathetic

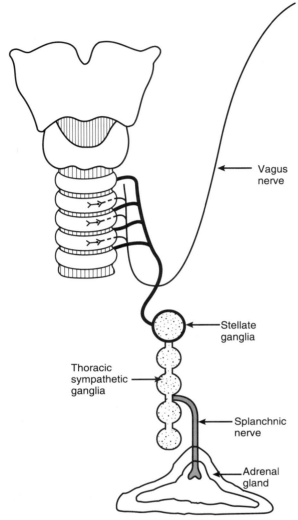

Figure 12–20. Efferent autonomic innervation of airways. A long preganglionic fiber carries efferent parasympathetic impulses to individual ganglia located in the subserosal portion of the airway. Postganglionic fibers are very short. Preganglionic sympathetic impulses are transmitted through the spinal column to a chain of ganglia located in the thorax. There are multiple synapses with each ganglion, and impulses may travel up and down the chain, thus amplifying the postganglionic response, which is transmitted globally to all organs through long postganglionic fibers. An extension of the chain, the greater splanchnic nerve, carries preganglionic impulses to the adrenal medulla, which is itself a large ganglion. The adrenal medulla secretes epinephrine directly into the systemic circulation. (From Leff AR, Munoz MN: Selective autonomic stimulation of canine trachealis with dimethylphenylpiperazinium. J Appl Physiol 51:428–437, 1981.)

nervous system causes generalized responses in multiple organ system. Efferent fibers originating in the central nervous system synapse initially in the sympathetic ganglia. The ganglia in the thoracic sympathetic chain influence the heart and lungs. Multiple ganglia are often involved in the response. In addition, each ganglion may initiate impulses in multiple postganglionic fibers, which then travel to multiple sites.

Adrenergic nerves that secrete norepinephrine directly innervate the mucous glands, blood vessels, and neural ganglia of airways. However, airway smooth muscle is not directly innervated by adrenergic nerves, and bronchomotor tone is not directly affected by sympathetic innervation. The adrenal medulla secretes epinephrine, which circulates in the bloodstream. Stimulated output of adrenal epinephrine has a bronchodilatory effect (e.g., during exercise).

Dopamine is a third catecholamine that is a naturally occurring neurotransmitter. It has no physiological function in the airways.

Nonadrenergic/Noncholinergic Inhibitory Innervation

The efferent nerves of the NANC inhibitory system course through the vagus nerve, and these fibers may share a common ganglion with parasympathetic fibers. Thus, they also have extremely short postganglionic segments. In contrast to the contractile response elicited in airway smooth muscle by parasympathetic nerves, NANC-inhibitory nerves cause relaxation of airway smooth muscle. The mediator of this response has not been identified, but it is likely a polypeptide(s) of small molecular weight.

The NANC system is so named because the mediator causing its response has not been identified but has been shown to be separate from the sympathetic and parasympathetic nervous systems. The response of the NANC-inhibitory system is anatomically as well as physiologically distinct from the NANC-stimulatory system (see earlier).

The afferent stimulus that activates the NANC-inhibitory system also has not been identified. Physical stimulation of the larynx causes activation of NANC fibers, and this causes bronchodilation. However, the homeostatic advantage of this response is unclear, and it is uncertain whether this represents the major action of the NANC-inhibitory system. Whatever the mediator(s) and/or mechanism of efferent NANC-inhibitory smooth muscle relaxation, the magnitude of the response can be substantial. The NANC-inhibitory system may also down-regulate the secretion of bronchoactive mediators from mast cells (see later). Further elucidation of its function will depend on identification of the mediator(s) causing airway smooth muscle relaxation.

Autonomic Organization in Airways

As outlined earlier there are at least four modes of innervation of conducting airways: (1) parasympathetic; (2) sympathetic; (3) NANC-inhibitory; and (4) NANC-stimulatory. Although it seems likely that the contractile systems (parasympathetic, NANC-stimulatory) would be counterbalanced by homeostatic impulses from the systems that relax airway smooth muscle (sympathetic, NANC-inhibitory) in normal individuals, this does not appear to occur.

It once was presumed that increases in parasympathetic (smooth muscle constrictor) tone in airways led to a compensatory increase in sympathetic tone, so that airway resistance would return toward normal in normal individuals. However, bronchoconstriction with a muscarinic agonist (i.e., a drug that causes increase in airways resistance) does not cause homeostatic secretion of catecholamine that would cause bronchodilation (Figure 12–21). Although abundant visceral sensory fibers affect airway tone by reflex conduction through the vagus nerve (see earlier), there is no sensor of airway caliber that results in alteration of sympathetic tone. Thus, bronchoconstriction does not stimulate the release of catecholamine, nor does it activate the NANC-inhibitory system.

Autonomic Regulation of Mast Cell Function

Under certain circumstances, mast cells in the airways release mediators that provoke an inflammatory response. In individuals with asthma, mast cell degranulation leads to bronchoconstriction. However, the chronic asthmatic state now is thought to be related more to the migration of inflammatory cells into the airway than to acute degranulation of respiratory mast cells.

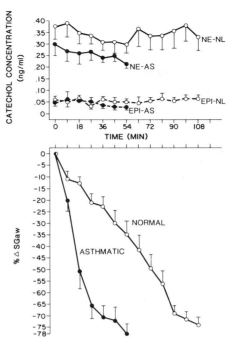

Figure 12–21. Effect of bronchoconstriction caused by an inhaled constrictor agonist (methacholine) on sympathetic secretion in human subjects. The agonist is given in progressively increased doses over time (abscissa); this causes a decrease in specific conductance of the airways (SGaw) in both normal and asthmatic humans, although asthmatics are more sensitive to bronchoconstriction. However, bronchoconstriction has no effect on blood concentration of either epinephrine (EPI) or norepinephrine (NE) in either normal (NL) or asthmatic (AS) individuals. These data indicate that there is no homeostatic proprioceptor that monitors airway caliber for sympathetic secretion. (From Sands MF, et al: Homeostatic regulation of bronchomotor tone by sympathetic activation during bronchoconstriction in normal and asthmatic humans. Am Rev Respir Dis 132:993–998, 1985.)

Both immune and non-immune-mediated mast cell secretion is mediated through a calcium ion–dependent intracellular process. Stimulation of the β-adrenergic receptor on the mast cell membrane causes activation of the enzyme adenylyl cyclase. This causes synthesis of cyclic 3'5'-adenosine monophosphate (AMP) from adenosine triphosphate (ATP). High intracellular concentrations of cyclic AMP lead to increases of intracellular calcium, and this results in partial or complete inhibition of mast cell synthesis and secretion of mediators (Figure 12–22). By contrast, stimulation of the α-adrenergic receptor causes inhibition of cyclic AMP synthesis

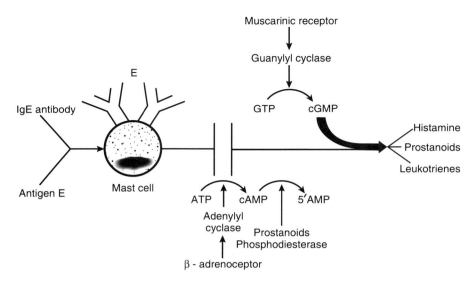

Figure 12–22. Regulation of mast cell secretion after immune activation. Bivalent linkage of IgE antibody to antigen E causes metabolic activation of the cell, and this results in secretion of the preformed mediator histamine and the immediate synthesis and secretion of other bronchoactive mediators (e.g., prostanoids and leukotrienes). Stimulation of the β-adrenergic receptor on the mast cell surface inhibits the process initiated by immune activation and reduces secretion. This is mediated by the membrane enzyme adenylyl cyclase, which converts adenosine triphosphate (ATP) to cyclic adenosine monophosphate (cAMP). An analogous system utilizing cyclic guanosine monophosphate (cGMP) causes augmentation of secretion.

and augmentation of mast cell secretion. Stimulation of the muscarinic receptor (parasympathomimetic stimulation) also causes augmentation of mast cell secretion. This results from synthesis of cyclic 3'5'-guanosine monophosphate (GMP), which causes increased concentration of intracellular calcium and augmented synthesis and secretion of mediators by the mast cell.

Experimental stimulation of the vagus nerve causes substantial augmentation of the mast cell response to immune stimulation in animals. Likewise, sympathetic stimulation causes complete inhibition of respiratory mast cell secretion. However, the homeostatic significance of these processes remains unclear, especially because changes in bronchomotor tone appear not to be linked between the parasympathetic and sympathetic nervous system (see Figure 12–21).

REGULATION OF TONE IN AIRWAY SMOOTH MUSCLE

Some degree of bronchomotor tone is maintained tonically by the parasympathetic nervous system through its direct innervation of airway smooth muscle. In normal individuals, administration of atropine or comparable muscarinic receptor blocking agents causes a reduction in airways resistance.

Sympathomimetic relaxing agents also relax actively contracted airway smooth muscle by stimulating the smooth muscle β-adrenergic receptor. Ultimately, smooth muscle tone is regulated by the availability of intercellular ionized calcium.

Contraction of airway smooth muscle is initiated either by voltage- or receptor-dependent calcium ion channels that reside on the surface membrane of airway smooth muscle. For example, increasing the concentration of potassium ion extracellularly causes membrane depolarization, and this opens voltage-dependent channels to calcium ions. The influx of calcium ions increases intracellular calcium availability, which activates actomyosin complexing (Figure 12–23). Thus, the active process of contraction is regulated by the availability of intracellular ionized calcium. Increasing concentrations of intracellular calcium cause activation of myosin ATPase, which causes phosphorylation of myosin light-chain. This phosphorylated form of myosin links with actin to generate contractile force. Decreasing calcium ion concentration inhibits myosin phosphorylation, and this causes relaxation.

Activation of the muscarinic receptor by parasympathetic stimulation causes activation of the polyphosphoinositide cascade shown in Figure 12–24. The "trigger" is the conversion of inositol *bis*-phosphate (IP$_2$) to the *tris*-phosphated (IP$_3$) form and the production of diacyl glyceride (DG) in the

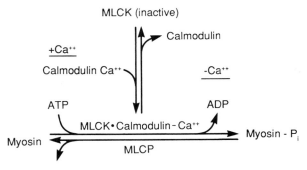

Figure 12-23. Activation of contraction. Inactive myosin light-chain kinase (MLCK) in the presence of calcium ion carried by calmodulin causes a complex by which myosin is phosphorylated (myosin-P_i). Phosphorylated myosin links with actin, and cross-bridge formation generates shortening of smooth muscle.

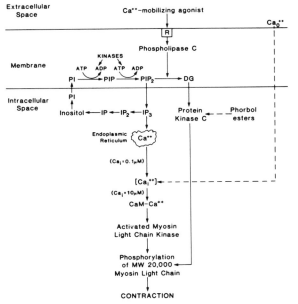

Figure 12-24. Activation of contraction of airway smooth muscle by stimulation of the muscarinic receptor (R). Binding to a membrane receptor activates inositol *bis*-phosphate (PIP_2) to the *tris*-phosphate (IP_3) form and diacyl glyceride (DG). IP_3 causes release of Ca^{2+} from the endoplasmic reticulum. Carried by calmodulin (CaM), this causes activation of myosin light-chain kinase (MLCK) (see Fig. 12-26). DG activates protein kinase C, which causes direct phosphorylation of myosin light-chain. (From Leff A: State of the art: Endogenous regulation of bronchomotor tone. Am Rev Respir Dis 137:1198-1216, 1988.)

membrane of the smooth muscle cell. Both IP_3 and DG cause mobilization of calcium from intracellular storage pools, and this promotes smooth muscle contraction by the mechanism outlined in Figure 12-23.

Relationship Between Airway Edema and Bronchomotor Tone

Under normal circumstances, resistance to airflow increases when smooth muscle constriction causes a narrowing of airway diameter. However, in certain inflammatory states there is fluid leak into the airway wall that causes airway wall edema. The associated swelling of the mucosa also causes airway narrowing and increased airflow resistance. There are two potential consequences of airway edema. First, the airway lumen may be narrowed, and this alone will increase airway resistance. Second, narrowing of the airway lumen will decrease the wall tension required to cause further narrowing. Thus, the same amount of smooth muscle tone will cause greater narrowing in an airway of smaller diameter than one of larger diameter. In this sense, narrowing begets further narrowing.

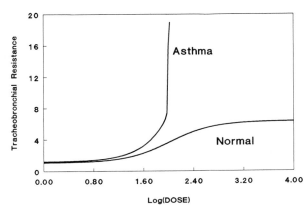

Figure 12-25. Theoretical response generated by computer model in an edematous asthmatic airway and a normal airway to a theoretical contractile agonist (e.g., methacholine). The tracheobronchial resistance to airflow increases to a point in normal persons, but then levels off—theoretically because tethering forces of the alveoli oppose further constriction of the airways. In contrast, there is an exponential increase in asthma airways because edema interferes with tethering forces. (From Leff AR: Toward the formation of a modern theory of asthma. Perspect Biol Med 33:292-302, 1990. Reproduced by permission of the University of Chicago Press.)

The edema fluid also may be deposited on the serosal side of the airway. If edema fluid is deposited external to the airway wall, it may interfere with tethering forces provided by surrounding lung parenchyma. Uncoupling of lung tethering forces may greatly augment contractile responses and lower the threshold stimulus to initiate bronchoconstriction. Interference with airway tethering structures also allows the airway to narrow without the "plateau response" observed under normal conditions (Figure 12–25).

DISTRIBUTION OF BRONCHOCONSTRICTOR RESPONSES

Maturational Changes in Bronchomotor Responses

In infants, bronchoconstrictor responses are weak. By 3 years of age, or sooner, these responses are substantial. The smooth muscle of juvenile airways is less responsive to a variety of contractile stimuli (Figure 12–26) in a number of species, and this may

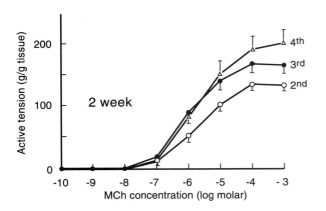
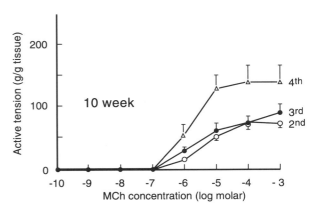
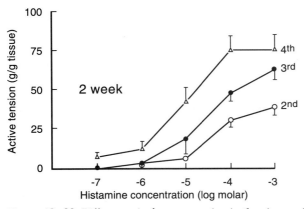
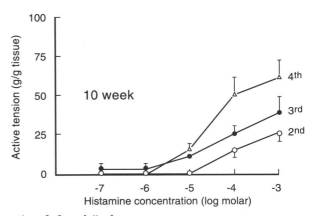

Figure 12–26. Differences in force generation in the airways (generations 2, 3, and 4) of a maturing animal. Contractile force is measured in vitro as active tension is measured isometrically. For both methacholine (MCh) and histamine there is an increase in contractile force in the more peripheral airway generations than in the more central airways, which decreased with maturation. (From Murphy TM, Roy L, Phillips IJ, Michell RW, Kelley EK, Munoz NM, Leff AR: Effect of maturation on topographical distribution of bronchoconstriction responses in large diameter airways of young swine. Am Rev Respir Dis 143:126–131, 1991.)

also be true for humans. The evolution of these changes in basal responsiveness to bronchoconstrictor stimuli that occurs with maturation is not yet understood.

Normal baseline airway resistance may be five times greater in children than in adults. This reflects largely differences in airway geometry and growth. As the airways grow, their diameters increase. This decreases baseline airway resistance and also decreases the response to bronchoconstrictor stimuli (the Laplace relationship; see Chapter 1).

Topographical Distribution of Airway Contractile Responses

A variety of opposing forces act on airways to influence their constriction, and these forces vary from airway generation to airway generation. The trachea (generation 0), mainstem (generation 1), and lobar (generation 2) airways are extraparenchymal (i.e., they are not tethered by the lung parenchyma). However, these airways contain rigid cartilage that opposes the narrowing of the airway as bronchomotor tone increases. Airways beyond generation 3 (segmental) bronchi are intraparenchymal and are therefore affected by lung interdependence forces that oppose bronchoconstriction. With each succeeding airway generation, the content of cartilage decreases, as does airway diameter. Both of these factors facilitate airway narrowing to a bronchoconstrictor stimulus. The decreased rigidity makes the airway more compressible. The decreased diameter facilitates airway narrowing (the law of Laplace).

Other factors are important in the topographical distribution of bronchoconstrictor response. The orientation of airway smooth muscle about the airway changes with each generation of airway. In the trachea, all of the airway smooth muscle is located in the posterior membrane. Contraction is opposed by the strong recoil of the cartilage. As the airway generations progress toward the periphery, the airway smooth muscle is wound progressively around the airway in a helical pattern, connecting the cartilaginous plates that become separate islands. The decreased rigidity and helical orientation of the airway smooth muscle favors more effective bronchoconstriction. Recent investigations have suggested that the ability of airway smooth muscle to generate contractile force also may increase with progressing airway generation (Figure 12–27).

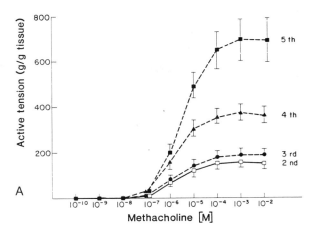

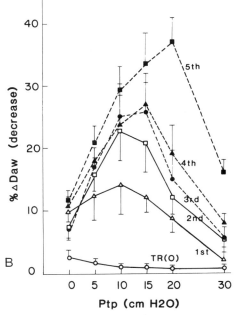

Figure 12–27. Differences in isometric force generation in the airway smooth muscle of excised airways stimulated with methacholine, a constrictor agonist. *A.* Generation 5 airways narrow much more than generation 2 or 3 airways. Length–tension curves generated in a living animal. Ordinate is the change in airway diameter measured radiographically, and abscissa is the transpulmonary pressure distending the airway. A length–tension relationship is obtained for each airway except the trachea. Note that at its optimal resting diameter, the fifth-generation airway narrows much more effectively than the first generation airway to the same stimulus. (*A,* from Shioya T, et al: Distribution of airway contractile response in major resistance airways of the lung. Am J Pathol 129:107–117, 1987; *B,* from Shioya T, et al: Effect of resting smooth muscle length on contractile responses in canine resistance airways in vivo. J Appl Physiol 62:711–717, 1987.)

How do all of these complex forces—some of which oppose each other—translate into airway narrowing in the living state? Despite substantial opposition from lung interdependence forces, parenchymal airways progressively narrow more effectively than more central airways to a variety of pharmacological stimuli. The initially narrower lumen, decreased rigidity, and greater force-generating capacity of the smooth muscle of these airways outweigh the distending force of the lung matrix that opposes contraction and tethers the airways open. The distribution of parasympathetic innervation is also substantially greater in the more central than in peripheral airways. This imparts greater constrictor tone on the central than on peripheral airways during physiological activation of the vagus nerve. Even so, peripheral airways narrow more effectively than do central airways during vagus nerve stimulation and for most other stimuli causing airway smooth muscle contraction.

Appendix

Review Questions and Answers

CHAPTER 1—Lung Mechanics: Statics

1. Under what circumstance are measurements of lung volume by the inert gas dilution technique likely to be inaccurate?

2. What lung volume is measured by body plethysmography to determine total lung capacity? Why is this volume used? What volume is added to it to obtain total lung capacity? How is the "added volume" obtained?

3. What factors determine the total lung capacity?

4. If a patient inspires to total lung capacity and the elastic recoil pressure is $+30$ cm H_2O, what are the P_{alv} and the P_{tp}?

5. What is the relative effect of low versus high lung volumes on effectiveness of pulmonary surfactant?

6. A patient inspires to total lung capacity, and the

P_{tp} is $+30$ cm H_2O (P_{alv} is zero; lung volume is stable). A shutter now is closed to form a sealed system between the alveolus and the mouth. The initial P_{pl} is -30 cm H_2O, but the patient now tries to exhale against the closed shutter and increases the P_{pl} to 100 cm H_2O. What effect does this have on P_{tp}?

7. What contributes to the additional work required to inflate a lung with air vs saline from residual volume to total lung capacity?

CHAPTER 2 — Lung Mechanics: Dynamics

1. How does a change in the radius of a tube alter the resistance to laminar flow?

2. Other factors remaining constant, how would an increase in the viscosity of a fluid influence the degree of turbulence under turbulent flow conditions?

3. Why is lung resistance greater than airways resistance?

4. What factors contribute to the decrease in airways resistance that occurs as lung volume is increased?

5. What factors would tend to increase maximal expiratory flow in the effort-independent region?

6. Why do small airways (<2 mm diameter) normally contribute so little to the overall airways resistance?

7. What flow regimens normally occur in the trachea? In bronchi less than 0.5 mm in diameter?

CHAPTER 3 — Ventilation

1. What are the principal muscles of inspiration? Of expiration?

2. Does ventilation cease if the phrenic nerve innervating the diaphragm is severed?

3. What is the inspired oxygen tension at the summit of Mt. Everest if the barometric pressure there is 250 torr?

4. What is the ambient oxygen tension in a hyperbaric diving chamber where the barometric pressure is 3800 torr and the oxygen dry gas fraction is 0.04?

5. Why is anatomical dead space ventilation smaller than physiological dead space ventilation?

6. Calculate the physiological dead space fraction if the P_{CO_2} in mixed expired gas is 27 torr while the P_{CO_2} in arterial blood is 40 torr.

7. Will an increase in minute ventilation produced by increasing respiratory frequency cause an equal increment in alveolar ventilation?

8. If the alveolar P_{CO_2} is found to be 60 torr in a patient breathing room air, what is a likely cause of this hypercapnia?

CHAPTER 4 — The Pulmonary Circulation

1. What might happen to the vertical gradient in blood flow in an individual in outer space under zero-gravity conditions?

2. If the left main pulmonary artery were transiently occluded and cardiac output remained unchanged (thus diverting all blood flow through the right lung), would the pulmonary artery pressure approximately double?

3. If the pulmonary artery pressure were reduced in a patient who had hemorrhaged, how might this influence the three zones of the lung?

4. What happens to fluid that leaks from the pulmonary capillaries into the lung interstitial space?

5. Why does the pulmonary vascular resistance increase at high lung volumes?

6. What effect might exposure to high altitude have on the pulmonary arterial pressure?

7. What are the different consequences of lung interstitial edema and alveolar edema for lung gas exchange?

8. What are the effective upstream and downstream pressures that determine blood flow in a lung region operating under zone II conditions?

CHAPTER 5 — Oxygen and Carbon Dioxide Transport in Blood

1. Calculate the oxygen content of arterial blood with a $P_{O_2} = 60$ torr, oxyhemoglobin saturation = 90%, and hemoglobin concentration = 14 g/dl.

2. What is the oxygen content of blood when the $P_{O_2} = 200$ torr and the hemoglobin concentration is 13 g/dl?

3. A patient taken from a burning building has a carboxyhemoglobin saturation of 20% and a hemoglobin concentration of 14 g/dl. How would this affect the arterial P_{O_2} and the arterial oxygen content?

4. If the normal hemoglobin concentration in blood could be doubled, could someone live normally if the arterial P_{O_2} was lowered to the point where arterial saturation was 50%?

5. Calculate the mixed venous blood oxygen content if the whole-body oxygen consumption is 250 ml/min, the cardiac output is 5 liters/min, and the arterial blood oxygen content is 20 ml/dl.

6. How does the uptake of oxygen along the pulmonary capillaries enhance the simultaneous elimination of carbon dioxide?

7. Why might a markedly left-shifted oxyhemoglobin dissociation curve (i.e., low hemoglobin P_{50}) be disadvantageous for oxygen transport in a subject living at sea level?

8. What is the significance of the oxygen tension, oxyhemoglobin saturation, and oxygen content in blood?

9. What roles does the hemoglobin molecule play in the transport of carbon dioxide from the tissues to the lungs?

CHAPTER 6 — Diffusion

1. If two gas volumes with different oxygen tensions are separated by a membrane, what effect will increasing the solubility of oxygen in a membrane have on the rate of equilibration between the compartments?

2. What processes contribute to the transport of gases from ambient air to the alveolar blood–gas membrane?

3. What are the components of the blood–gas barrier?

4. Is the transport of oxygen in pulmonary capillaries normally limited by perfusion or diffusion?

5. What factors might contribute to a decrease in the diffusing capacity measurement for carbon monoxide?

6. How does exercise affect the carbon monoxide diffusing capacity measurement?

7. Blood with a P_{O_2} of 50 torr (oxygen content, 16 ml/dl) is separated from a reservoir of saline whose P_{O_2} is 500 torr (oxygen content, 1.5 ml/dl) by a gas-permeable membrane. In which direction will the oxygen diffuse?

8. Why is the diffusing capacity for oxygen difficult to measure experimentally?

CHAPTER 7 — Ventilation–Perfusion Relationships

1. What is the significance of the calculated ideal alveolar oxygen tension for a lung?

2. Why does systemic arterial blood P_{O_2} decrease more than arterial P_{CO_2} increases when shunt or ventilation–perfusion inequality is present?

3. What can be done to improve the arterial oxygen tension and content in a lung with a 25% shunt?

4. Why doesn't ventilation with pure oxygen correct the hypoxemia caused by shunt?

5. When an alveolus fills with edema fluid, does any gas exchange occur in that alveolus?

6. What factors determine the alveolar P_{O_2} in a single alveolus?

7. Why is the $(A-a)D_{O_2}$ greater than 0 torr in a normal healthy lung?

8. Do alveoli near the base of a normal vertical lung exhibit higher or lower $\dot{V}_A/\dot{Q}$ ratios than alveoli near the apex?

CHAPTER 8 — Control of Ventilation

1. Why do skin divers hyperventilate prior to diving?

2. Which chemoreceptors mediate the ventilatory response to hypoxia?

3. Which chemoreceptors mediate the ventilatory response to carbon dioxide?

4. What factors can depress the ventilatory response to carbon dioxide?

5. What factors determine the pH in the cerebrospinal fluid?

6. What effect would vagal nerve cold-block (to block nerve conduction reversibly) have on the resting ventilatory pattern?

7. What ventilatory pattern would result if the spinal column were sectioned at the caudal end of the medulla?

CHAPTER 9 — Physiology of Exercise

1. Which form of metabolism most efficiently utilizes glucose stores — aerobic or anaerobic? What is the significance of this in endurance exercise (e.g., marathon running)?

2. What is the significance of aerobic versus anaerobic metabolism in short-term maximal exercise (e.g., high jumping)?

3. Which factors limit maximal exercise?

4. During exercise the respiratory quotient increases from 0.85 to about 1.0 near anaerobic threshold. What are the consequences of this for alveolar ventilation? What is the mechanism of this effect?

5. At anaerobic threshold, what changes occur in minute ventilation? What is the mechanism?

CHAPTER 10 — Lung Growth and Development

1. During pregnancy, there is a 15% to 40% (depending on the stage) increase in the cardiac output of the mother. What is the functional advantage of this to the fetus?

2. Describe the prenatal and postnatal functions of the foramen ovale and ductus arteriosus? What problems are likely to result if these structures remain patent (open) after birth.

3. Describe differences in the oxygen content–oxygen tension curves of the fetus and the mother. What accounts for this?

4. What is the P_{O_2} of blood in the umbilical vein? How is the fetus able to survive and grow with this arterial P_{O_2}?

5. At birth there are no alveoli. How is the neonate, which now must breathe air, able to survive?

CHAPTER 11 — Lung Defenses

1. If a load of airborne particles with a 20-μm average diameter is inhaled, where will most of these particles be trapped?

2. What is the primary mechanism responsible for clearance of particulate debris from the alveolar space?

3. What mechanisms are available for removal of hydrogen peroxide?

4. What mechanisms are available for the clearance of hydroxyl free radicals?

5. What mechanisms contribute to the clearance of superoxide anion?

6. What factors determine the likelihood that hyperoxic lung damage will occur in a patient breathing enriched inspired oxygen?

7. From which region of the lung are trapped particles cleared most slowly?

CHAPTER 12 — Biology of Conducting Airways

1. Describe the change in function and corresponding morphological changes in the airway epithelium beginning in the upper airways and terminating in the alveoli.

2. List the major components of the autonomic nervous system innervating the conducting airways. What function does each system serve?

3. What changes occur in the response of the airways of the lung to bronchoconstrictor stimuli as children mature to adulthood? What is the mechanism of these changes?

4. How does contraction of airway smooth muscle differ from skeletal muscle?

5. During deep inspiration, the airways dilate. What neural mechanism contributes to this response?

6. What factors affect the ability of extraparenchymal airways to narrow? What factors affect the intraparenchymal airways? Which shorten most effectively? Why?

7. It has been hypothesized that edema in peribronchial airways (the region of the lung surrounding the airway) may augment contraction to bronchoconstrictor stimuli in certain inflammatory states, such as human asthma. How might this occur?

ANSWERS

CHAPTER 1—Lung Mechanics: Statics

1. The gas dilution technique is inaccurate whenever there is substantial maldistribution of ventilation caused by obstructed airways. This results in noncommunicating spaces in which the inert gas is not diluted. The concentration of expired gas after "equilibration" thus is greater than it would be if there were adequate distribution of the gas.

2. The gas volume typically measured is the functional residual capacity (FRC). This is a highly reproducible volume (one comes to this volume at the end of each breath), and it is a comfortable volume at which to pant. FRC can be added to inspiratory capacity determined by spirometry to give total lung capacity.

3. Total lung capacity is determined by the ability of the respiratory muscles to oppose the recoil of the lung and chest wall. At TLC, both the lung and chest wall recoil toward lesser lung volumes. To increase lung volume, the inspiratory muscles must shorten, and as they shorten, they move to a less favorable portion of the length-tension curve. Thus, with increasing lung volume, respiratory muscles generate less force. When the recoil of the lung and chest wall is equivalent to the maximal (progressively decreasing) force that the respiratory muscles can generate, TLC is determined.

4. Assuming that lung volume is not changing, P_{tp} is $+30$ cm H_2O; that is, the distending force equals the recoil force. Because lung volumes are not changing, there is no pressure gradient between the open glottis and the alveoli) and alveolar pressure is zero.

5. Pulmonary surfactant has its greatest surface tension reducing effect at low lung volumes.

6. The P_{tp} is unchanged. $P_{tp} = P_{alv} - P_{pl}$. If P_{pl} increases from -30 to $+100$ cm H_2O, this increase of 130 cm H_2O is transmitted to the alveolus. The P_{alv}, which initially was zero, now is 130 $(30 + 100)$ cm H_2O, and P_{pl} is 100 cm H_2O. Thus $P_{alv} - P_{pl}$ remains the same ($+30$ cm H_2O).

7. The surface tension that must be overcome when there is an air–liquid interface.

CHAPTER 2—Lung Mechanics: Dynamics

1. Changes in the resistance are inversely proportional to changes in the radius raised to the fourth power.

2. Increasing the viscosity would reduce the Reynolds number, thereby reducing the degree of turbulence.

3. Airways resistance is a component of lung resistance, which also includes a component from lung viscous resistance.

4. Increased airway wall tethering augments the caliber of the airways, tending to reduce airways resistance. In addition, there is a decrease in airway smooth muscle constriction caused by a decrease in parasympathetic nervous system tone. This is an autonomic reflex response mediated by stretch receptors in the lung tissue near the alveoli.

5. Increases in lung static recoil, increases in the stiffness of the airways, and decreases in airway resistance will tend to augment flow-limited exhalation.

6. Because the number of small airways in parallel is large relative to their individual resistances, they normally contribute little to airways resistance.

7. Airflow in the trachea is fully turbulent, even in quiet breathing. Flow regimens in very small airways approach laminar flow conditions.

CHAPTER 3—Ventilation

1. The major muscles of inspiration are the diaphragm and the external intercostal muscles. The principal muscles of expiration are the abdominal wall muscles and the internal intercostals, although expiration is normally passive at rest.

2. No, because ventilation can be maintained by the intercostal muscles and the accessory muscles, which are innervated by spinal motor nerves.

3. Inspired air is warmed to body temperature and saturated with water vapor, so the inspired $P_{O_2} = (250 - 47) \cdot 0.2093 = 42.5$ torr.

4. Assuming the gas is dry in the chamber, $P_{O_2} = 3800 \cdot 0.04 = 152$ torr.

5. Physiological dead space includes ventilation to the conducting airways (anatomical dead space) plus any extra ventilation that is used to overventilate some alveoli.

6. Physiological dead space will be $1.0 - (27/40) = 0.33$ or 33%.

7. No, because some of the increase in ventilation contributes to an increase in anatomical dead space ventilation.

8. The increased arterial P_{CO_2} must be caused by an increased alveolar P_{CO_2} resulting from inadequate alveolar ventilation relative to the metabolic production of carbon dioxide. This is termed hypoventilation.

CHAPTER 4—The Pulmonary Circulation

1. In the absence of gravity, the distribution of blood flow from the top to the bottom of the lung should become more uniform.

2. No. Any increase in the pulmonary arterial pressure will recruit and distend vessels in the right lung, tending to reduce their resistance. Pressure may increase but should not double.

3. A sufficient decrease in mean pulmonary arterial pressure could cause zone I regions to appear at the uppermost regions of the lung. A decrease in pulmonary venous pressure could also convert zone III regions into zone II regions.

4. Most fluid that leaves the vascular space is eventually returned to the circulation through the lymphatic system.

5. Stretch and distortion of alveolar septal walls causes an increase in the resistance of alveolar vessels, including alveolar capillaries.

6. Exposure to high altitude causes the alveolar oxygen tension to decrease. This can cause acute hypoxic pulmonary vasoconstriction in all lung regions, causing an increase in pulmonary arterial pressure. This effect is reversed on return to sea level.

7. Interstitial edema has less of an influence on lung gas exchange because it does not significantly interfere with gas transfer between alveolar gas and pulmonary capillary blood. By contrast, in alveolar edema the flooded alveoli cannot participate in gas exchange yet still receive blood flow.

8. Local pulmonary arterial pressure and local alveolar hydrostatic pressure determine blood flow in zone II.

CHAPTER 5—Oxygen and Carbon Dioxide Transport in Blood

1. Blood oxygen content = hemoglobin-bound component + dissolved oxygen components:

Oxygen content (ml/dl)

$$= (1.39 \text{ ml/g})(14 \text{ g/dl})(0.90)$$

$$+ (0.003 \text{ ml/(dl} \cdot \text{torr}))(60 \text{ torr})$$

$$= 17.51 + 0.18 = 17.69 \text{ ml/dl}.$$

2. Blood oxygen content = hemoglobin-bound component + dissolved oxygen components:

Oxygen content (ml/dl)

$$= (1.39 \text{ ml/g})(13 \text{ g/dl})(1.0)$$

$$+ (0.003 \text{ ml/(dl} \cdot \text{torr}))(200 \text{ torr}) = 18.07 + 0.60$$

$$= 18.67 \text{ ml/dl}.$$

[Recall that hemoglobin is fully saturated at a P_{O_2} of 200 torr.]

3. Arterial blood oxygen content would be reduced because 20% of the binding sites for oxygen would be occupied by carbon monoxide molecules. Arterial P_{O_2} would not be affected, since this is determined by the partial pressure of oxygen in blood.

4. Probably not. The diffusion of oxygen out of capillary blood into the systemic tissues is set by the oxygen tension difference between capillary blood and the surrounding tissue. If arterial P_{O_2} is abnormally low, the capillary partial pressure gradient driving oxygen diffusion into the tissues may not be adequate to maintain normal metabolic activity, even if the blood oxygen content is normal.

5. Oxygen consumption ($\dot{V}_{O_2}$) is the product of the cardiac output and the arteriovenous oxygen content difference. Hence:

$$250 \text{ ml/min} = (50 \text{ dl/min})(20 \text{ ml/dl}$$

$$- \text{ mixed venous oxygen content})$$

$$\text{Mixed venous oxygen content} = 15 \text{ ml/dl}$$

[Note that 5 liters/min = 50 dl/min.]

6. The uptake of oxygen shifts the carbon dioxide content–partial pressure relationship downward. This allows a greater decrease in carbon dioxide content along the pulmonary capillary for a given difference between mixed venous and end-capillary P_{CO_2}.

7. If arterial blood hemoglobin saturation is virtually complete, a left-shifted dissociation curve necessitates a lower average tissue capillary P_{O_2} to maintain a given arteriovenous oxygen content difference. This lowers the partial pressure gradient driving diffusion of oxygen out of the systemic capillaries.

8. Saturation reflects the percentage of the hemoglobin binding sites that are occupied by oxygen; oxygen tension reflects the driving gradient for oxygen to enter or leave the blood and is proportional to the dissolved component of oxygen content. Oxygen content is a measure of the volume of oxygen contained in a unit of blood, which is the sum of dissolved and hemoglobin-bound contributions.

9. Hemoglobin binds carbon dioxide directly as carbamino compounds. It also buffers the hydrogen ions released as bicarbonate formed in the red cells, promoting additional carbon dioxide carrying capacity.

CHAPTER 6 — Diffusion

1. Increasing the solubility in the membrane will speed up the rate of equilibration.

2. Convection carries air from the mouth to the distal airways; diffusion transports gas up to the blood–gas barrier.

3. Traveling from the alveolus toward the capillary: surfactant layer, alveolar epithelium, interstitial space, and pulmonary capillary endothelium. On average, this barrier is about 0.5 μm in thickness.

4. Oxygen equilibration is normally limited by perfusion, because blood equilibrates with alveolar gas before the end of the pulmonary capillary.

5. Decreased surface area, increased membrane thickness, decreased blood hemoglobin concentration, or abnormally increased blood carboxyhemoglobin levels.

6. By increasing the number of perfused capillaries and the volume of blood within alveolar septal capillaries, exercise increases the diffusing capacity for carbon monoxide.

7. Oxygen will diffuse from the region of higher partial pressure to lower partial pressure.

8. The $D_{L_{O_2}}$ is difficult to measure because the average difference in P_{O_2} between alveolar gas and capillary blood cannot be measured. Thus, the average driving gradient for diffusion is unknown.

CHAPTER 7 — Ventilation–Perfusion Relationships

1. The value calculated from the ideal alveolar oxygen equation represents the highest blood P_{O_2} value that could be produced by a given lung. Thus, the $(A-a)D_{O_2}$ represents the difference between what the lung theoretically could produce and what it actually yielded.

2. When shunt or ventilation–perfusion inequality is present, blood from normally ventilated alveoli admixes with blood from nonventilated (or poorly ventilated) lung regions. Because the oxygen partial pressure–content relationship is sigmoidal, excessive ventilation of normal alveoli cannot significantly augment the oxygen content in the blood leaving them. Because the partial pressure–content relationship for carbon dioxide is much more linear, excessive ventilation of some alveoli can effectively compensate for the underventilation of others, in terms of carbon dioxide exchange. This difference is often manifested by a low arterial P_{O_2} with a normal P_{CO_2} in many forms of lung disease.

3. Increasing the inspired oxygen concentration and increasing the mixed venous oxygen content will increase both the systemic arterial blood P_{O_2} and content if the shunt remains constant.

4. Ventilation with pure oxygen cannot fully correct the hypoxemia caused by shunt because the nonventilated lung regions cannot be directly affected by a gas that does not ventilate them.

5. Flooded alveoli do not participate in gas exchange because ventilation cannot enter the alveolus. In theory, some oxygen might diffuse through the edema fluid to reach the capillary, but in practice this does not occur to a significant extent.

6. Alveolar P_{O_2} is determined by the inspired oxygen tension, the mixed venous oxygen tension, and the ventilation–perfusion ratio.

7. Even healthy lungs exhibit a small $(A-a)D_{O_2}$ that is caused largely by small topograpical ventilation–perfusion heterogeneity, which arises from the effects of gravity on the distributions of ventilation and blood flow.

8. Because they are better perfused than ventilated, alveoli near the bottom of the lung exhibit lower $\dot{V}_A/\dot{Q}$ ratios than those near the top.

CHAPTER 8—Control of Ventilation

1. Voluntary hyperventilation reduces the alveolar P_{CO_2} and increases alveolar P_{O_2}. This delays the eventual increase in P_{CO_2} and decrease in P_{O_2} that forces the diver to return to the surface. Breath-holding duration is limited by the point where automatic ventilatory control dominates the control of inspiratory muscle motor neurons.

2. The ventilatory response to hypoxia is mediated exclusively by the peripheral chemoreceptors.

3. Ventilatory responses to carbon dioxide are mediated by the peripheral chemoreceptors (approximately 40%) and by the medullary chemoreceptors (approximately 60%).

4. Anesthetic agents, narcotics, barbiturates, and other central nervous system depressants can reduce the ventilatory response to carbon dioxide.

5. The pH in cerebrospinal fluid is influenced by the ratio of the bicarbonate concentration to the P_{CO_2}.

6. Vagal cold block would have a minimal effect on the pattern of ventilation in an adult because the Hering-Breuer reflex contributes minimally to the determination of resting tidal volume.

7. Apnea would result.

CHAPTER 9—Physiology of Exercise

1. Aerobic metabolism produces 36 moles of adenosine triphosphate (ATP) for each mole of glucose metabolized, while only two ATP equivalents are produced by anaerobic metabolism of glucose. Thus, glucose utilization is 18-fold more efficient under aerobic conditions. During endurance exercise such as marathon running, this is important because glucose stores are limited. If there is a higher threshold for anaerobic metabolism, these limited stores will be utilized more slowly and stores of glucose will be preserved. At high levels of exercise, glucose is the predominant substrate that is metabolized.

2. Anaerobic threshold is not a factor in high jumping, which requires a burst of activity but no endurance. Fast-twitch fibers, which have a relatively low anaerobic threshold, may be particularly useful in providing the "spring" to clear the bar.

3. In health, the limiting factors of maximal exercise are the heart rate and stroke volume of the left ventricle of the heart (i.e., the cardiac output). These factors determine the amount of oxygen that can be delivered to the muscles during maximal exercise. Exercise is never limited by pulmonary gas exchange in normal persons.

4. As the amount of oxygen consumption increases, the carbon dioxide production also increases. To maintain a constant arterial blood pH of 7.40, carbon dioxide must be eliminated at the same rate at which it is being produced. This requires a proportionate increase in minute ventilation. Note that as the respiratory quotient increases, the relative amount of carbon dioxide production increases as well, and a further increment in minute ventilation is necessary to preserve that pH of 7.40. Note that this pH is no longer preserved above the anaerobic threshold.

5. At anaerobic threshold, lactic acidosis causes respiratory chemoreceptor stimulation and there is a disproportionate increase in minute ventilation (see Figure 9–8) above the linear increase that has occurred from rest to anaerobic threshold. This occurs in two stages. During the stage of isocapnic buffering there is a "sluggish" ventilatory response to acidosis and the arterial blood pH decreases. Within about 2 minutes, a "steeper" response occurs (see Figure 9–8), as progressive decreases in pH further stimulate ventilation. Note that anaerobic threshold occurs only at about 50% of the maximal exercise capacity ($\dot{V}_{O_2}$max).

CHAPTER 10—Lung Growth and Development

1. The metabolic demands of the fetus are very large—above twice that per body weight of the adult. There is rapid growth and development, which requires sustained delivery of nutrients and oxygen to the fetus. By increasing cardiac output, the mother can meet these requirements. Note that an increased cardiac output is a virtual physiological necessity. The "anemia" of pregnancy itself reduces the oxygen-carrying capacity of maternal blood to the uterus for placental oxygen exchange.

2. Before birth, the foramen ovale and ductus arteriosus are the conduits through which blood is diverted past the lungs to the systemic circulation. Because the lungs are not exchanging gas in utero, the blood does not need to pass through the lungs. The circulation is distributed to developing organs through the systemic circulation. After birth, the neonate rapidly must become an air-breathing organism. To do this, the lungs must expand, and all blood must pass through the lungs before entering the systemic circulation. If the foramen ovale and ductus arteriosus do not close, the systemic blood pressure, which is higher than the pulmonary blood pressure, will cause a huge increase in pulmonary blood flow. Blood entering the aorta will again be pumped back into the right side of the heart and diverted away from the systemic circulation. In life, the foramen ovale closes soon after birth because the decrease in pulmonary arterial blood pressure causes it to close. A short period of time after birth, the ductus arteriosus also closes. When this does not occur, surgery is required to ligate the ductus.

3. Figure 10–3 shows the difference in these curves. Because the fetus has a greater blood hemoglobin concentration, the maximal carrying capacity for oxygen per deciliter of blood is greater than that for the mother. Hence the maximum point on the curve is greater (about 20 mg/dl for the fetus versus 15 mg/dl for the mother). The fetal hemoglobin also has a lesser P_{50} than the maternal (20 torr for the fetus versus 27 torr for the mother), thus, at an oxygen tension of 20 torr, the fetal arterial blood is 75% saturated.

4. The P_{O_2} is no more than 30 torr. The shape of the oxygen dissociation curve (Figure 10–3) reveals that substantial unloading of oxygen to the tissues is thus possible at this low tension. See also discussion to question 3 above.

5. Gas exchange occurs through respiratory ducts and terminal saccules. The final architecture of the lung is not complete for at least 7 years after birth, and there is substantial growth of the adult-configured lung from age 7 to maturation. In short, gas exchange does not require alveoli per se; the function of alveoli is served by precursor anatomical structures.

CHAPTER 11—Lung Defenses

1. Most particles of this size will become trapped in the nasopharynx and the conducting airways.

2. Alveolar macrophages remove material from the alveoli.

3. Catalase is an enzyme that degrades hydrogen peroxide into water and oxygen.

4. The hydroxyl radical is extremely reactive and oxidizes nearby molecules virtually instantaneously. Hence, the available concentration of hydroxyl radical is very small. Nonenzymatic scavengers contribute to the removal of radicals generated by the hydroxyl radical.

5. Superoxide anion can be degraded enzymatically by superoxide dismutase or scavenged by nonenzymatic pathways.

6. The higher the inspired oxygen concentration and the longer the duration of exposure, the greater the probability that hyperoxic lung injury will occur.

7. Trapped particles are cleared most slowly from the interstitial space.

CHAPTER 12—Biology of Conducting Airways

1. The epithelium of the trachea is pseudostratifed and columnar. It forms tight junctions to prevent entry of solutes and particulates. This epithelium also has cilia, which sweep trapped particulates and potentially infectious organisms out of the lung. There is a gradual transition in the epithelium toward the alveoli. At the alveolar level, the epithelium consists of three cell types. Type I cells cover most of the area. They are flat and thin and contain no cilia. They closely approximate the capillaries of the pulmonary circulation and are ideally designed for gas exchange. Type II cells secrete surfactant, which is not synthesized by the epithelium of the

large airways. Type III cells have a more obscure function and are minority constituents.

2. There are four:

a. The parasympathetic nervous system. These nerves originate in the brain stem and have very long preganglionic fibers. The very short postganglionic fibers are in the organs they innervate, permitting selective stimulation of individual organs. The neurotransmitter is acetylcholine.

b. The sympathetic nervous system. This system has two components: (1) direct innervation (neurotransmitter: norepinephrine) and (2) adrenal secretion (hormone: epinephrine). The nerves that innervate the airways arise from thoracic sympathetic ganglia and have long postganglionic fibers. They innervate mucus glands and facilitate the "watery" component of mucus secretion. Sympathetic nerves do not innervate directly the airway smooth muscle. The adrenal gland secretes epinephrine, which reaches the airways through the systemic circulation. Epinephrine causes airway smooth muscle relaxation, but this is probably not a significant physiological effect except during exercise. Note that the ganglia of the sympathetic nervous system connect to each other (see Figure 12–20) and are designed for a "flight and fright" response (i.e., general activation that is nonspecific for many organs). There are as many as 20 synapses in each ganglion, and many organs are thus activated at once.

c. The nonadrenergic/noncholinergic (NANC) inhibitory system. Little is known about this system. These fibers, which inhibit airway smooth muscle tone, travel with the vagus nerve, but, unlike the parasympathetic nervous system, NANC-activation causes bronchodilation. The transmitter is unknown.

d. The NANC-stimulatory system. These nerves are sensory fibers that secrete antidromally. The transmitters are believed to be substance P and neurokinin A. They cause airway smooth muscle contraction and edema. Activation occurs in asthmatic humans during hyperventilation or airway cooling.

3. The airway resistance decreases substantially. This is believed to result from growth of conducting airways, which increases the diameter of the airways and reduces baseline lung resistance. The initial larger diameter of the airways also reduces the response of adult airways to bronchoconstrictor stimuli. Recent investigations also have suggested that there are maturation changes in airway smooth muscle responses to bronchoconstrictor stimuli as well. Both of these factors may explain why some asthmatic children "outgrow" their disease.

4. Airway smooth muscle is not striated, has no Z-bands, and consists of discrete sarcomeres. Airway smooth muscle does not generate action potentials. Compared with skeletal muscle, airway smooth muscle contracts and relaxes very slowly and peak tensions may not be reached until 10 to 12 seconds after a maximal stimulus. Airway smooth muscle can also generate force at resting length substantially below its optimal point on the length-tension curve. Thus, airway smooth muscle can shorten much more than skeletal muscle.

5. The alveolar stretch receptors are activated. This inhibits vagal tone at the central nervous system level. This reduces parasympathetic constrictor tone on the airways, and they dilate.

6. Narrowing of the extraparenchymal airways is limited largely by the rigidity of the supporting cartilage and the ability of the smooth muscle to overcome that recoil. For the intraparenchymal airways, the cartilage is less rigid, but these airways are tethered open by the connections to the surrounding lung (the lung interdependence forces). In general, a fifth- or sixth-generation airway will narrow more than a first- or second-generation airway. The amount of airway smooth muscle in both is about the same. Apparently, the larger diameter and rigidity of the cartilage in the more proximal airways impose a greater limitation to airway narrowing than does the tethering effect of the lung.

7. Theoretically, edema could interfere with the tethering effects that pull the airway open. The airway then is free to narrow in unopposed fashion. This would both lower the threshold and augment the maximal constriction of a contracting airway.

Index

Note: Page numbers in *italics* indicate illustrations. Page numbers followed by (t) refer to tables.